Primary Prevention for Children and Families

The *Journal of Children in Contemporary Society* series:

- *Young Children in a Computerized Environment*
- *Primary Prevention for Children & Families*
- *The Puzzling Child: From Recognition to Treatment*
- *Children of Exceptional Parents*
- *Childhood Depression*

Primary Prevention for Children and Families

Mary Frank, MS in Education, Editor

Journal of Children in Contemporary Society
Volume 14, Numbers 2/3

The Haworth Press
New York

The Haworth Press, Inc., 28 East 22 Street, New York, NY 10010

Library of Congress Cataloging in Publication Data
Main entry under title:

Primary prevention for children & families.

    (Journal of children in contemporary society ; v. 14, no. 2/3)
    Bibliography: p.
    1. Child psychopathology—Prevention. 2. Community mental health services. 3. Child mental health services.
I. Frank, Mary (Isabelle) II. Series.
RJ499.P714   362.2'0425   81-17858
ISBN 0-86656-107-2   AACR2

Primary Prevention
for Children and Families

Journal of Children in Contemporary Society
Volume 14, Numbers 2/3

CONTENTS:

INTRODUCTION

Since the growing field of primary prevention of mental disorders is currently having an impact on promoting innovative changes within communities to provide intervention and treatment of its children, to its families, and to its elderly, this issue was designed to review the present state of the art as it pertains to children and families. This will be of value to social scientists, to other professionals, and to students in the human sciences.

The contributors for this issue were selected because they have made significant contributions to the field. Collectively, they have reviewed its historical origins, stated strategies which would further revolutionize the field, identified intervention strategies that support children and families, presented a model that can be used to target populations at risk, presented models that can be utilized to bring about healthy environmental climates, presented a theoretical framework for educating practitioners in primary prevention, and presented a model for training practitioners who are presently in the field. The concluding article states the present and future status of the National Institute of Mental Health Prevention Program, the federal agency that supports much of the ongoing development of primary prevention in this country.

This is the first issue in a series of four mental health monographs. It is first because it establishes a foundation and a need for prevention, intervention, and treatment of the problems that will be discussed in the succeeding issues. These will be: "The Puzzling Child: From Recognition to Treatment," "Children of Exceptional Parents," and "Childhood Depression."

1

The Editor and Associate Editor are grateful to the theme consultants who gave much deliberate thought to the components of primary prevention which best describe the field as it relates to children and families. They are, also, grateful to the contributors who responded with articles that are theoretical as well as highly pragmatic in nature.

MIF

HISTORICAL OVERVIEW

A BRIEF HISTORICAL PERSPECTIVE ON THE PRIMARY PREVENTION OF CHILDHOOD MENTAL DISORDERS

George W. Albee, PhD

ABSTRACT. A synopsis and overview of the history of primary prevention is presented with special attention to the prevention of emotional problems of children. The need for new models for disorders is considered and the implications of a new model that is shown can lead to revolutionary changes in the whole mental health field.

A serious concern with efforts at preventing mental and emotional disturbances in children clearly is *not* a universal human phenomenon. The human animal has been selected over two or three million years of evolution to care for and nurture its helpless offspring—those who were not nurturant lost their infants and their "nurture genes." Defense and protection of the helpless young is an obvious behavior among mammals, as any farmer or zoologist can attest. But it is largely among the relatively self-conscious, advantaged, and empathic societies that there exists a deliberate concern for the emotional security of young children as a preventive effort against later mental disorders.

A high birth rate and high rate of infant and child mortality has been characteristic of most human societies from the eons of pre-civilization food-gathering nomadic groups through the pre-industrial agrarian era.

Dr. George Albee is Professor of Psychology, University of Vermont, Burlington, VT 05405.

Only recently have public health methods sharply reduced infant and child mortality throughout the world and, in the absence of changes in conception rate, led to the enormous explosion in the populations of the industrially underdeveloped countries of the world. The uncertainty of survival and the grinding poverty in much of the contemporary world makes a concern with primary prevention of childhood emotional distress a luxury most societies cannot afford, or even think much about.

The present century has witnessed an enormously expanded concern in the United States (and in other relatively affluent societies) with effective methods of improving public health. The success of public health methods is responsible for dramatic increases in longevity, in reduced infant and child mortality, and in reduction in the complications of pregnancy and the mortality of women in childbirth. The development of effective preventive and treatment approaches to the infectious diseases that have long plagued humankind, and the recent development of effective methods of contraception, all combine to change the earlier fatalism that characterized attitudes toward the survival of children, especially in the industrializing societies of the world.

Understandably, public health approaches and methods with clear-cut validity in preventing infectious diseases have influenced the thinking of professionals concerned with attempts at preventing ''mental illness,'' including mental and emotional disturbances in children. A more detailed account of this complex field of primary prevention is available, with a lengthy list of references in Kessler and Albee (1975), and Albee and Joffe (1977). In brief, prevention efforts in the field of mental health have borrowed from public health the strategies of (1) eliminating the noxious agent (examples: reducing stress, genetic counseling), (2) strengthening the host (examples: building social competence and coping skills, raising self-esteem, and developing support groups), and (3) preventing noxious agents from reaching the host (examples: foster home care, day-care, removing salt and sugar from baby foods).

Prevention efforts did not begin at one time and one place. An attempt to trace all the converging streams is beyond the space limit of this brief paper (see suggested readings) but a few relevant contributions, and controversies, deserve attention.

At the core of efforts at primary prevention is the question of the modifiability of individual human personality development as a consequence of manipulable human experience. While the choice of models is not either-or, one current ideology views development as relatively rigid—an unfolding of preprogrammed stages fixed in a biological blueprint laid down in genetic, biochemical, and neurological templates that are more or less invulnerable to experience. This view emphasizes the role of heredity, for example, in the causation of "mental illness" and mental retardation, and stresses such preventive efforts as genetic counseling, amniocentesis leading to therapeutic abortion, sterilization of the retarded and the insane, chemical correction of physical imbalances, etc. In direct contrast is an alternative ideology that views disturbed human behavior as resulting largely from socially learned patterns of human interaction and reactions to external stress. This latter view, more common among educators and psychotherapists, emphasizes the prevention of faulty interpersonal learning and the acquisition of coping skills in reducing stress and in enhancing the satisfaction of interpersonal relations. The first view is well illustrated by the statement of psychiatrists Lamb and Zusman (1978) that: "Mental illness is probably in large part genetically determined and it is probably therefore not preventable, at most only modifiable. Even that it can be modified is questioned by many and there is little hard evidence one way or the other" (p. 13). The polar opposite social learning view is increasingly expressed (Albee, 1979, 1980); over the past half dozen years a well-documented record of evidence for the effectiveness of primary prevention programs has been accumulated (see, for example, Albee and Joffe, 1977 on the issues; Kent and Rolf, 1979 on building social competence in children and Joffe and Bond, 1981 on facilitating infant and early childhood development).

The hypothesis has long been held that different patterns of child rearing, each consistently followed, result in significant differences in later mental health of children and adults. Freud's efforts at alleviating adult distress through psychoanalysis inevitably led him back to the childhood experiences of his clients. While Freud never made explicit his attitudes toward emotional prophylaxis (see Lemkau, 1956) still many of his followers, including his daughter, Anna Freud, have discussed the importance of controlling childhood experience with a view to promoting later mental health and maturity. Similarly Alfred Adler has written extensively about the relation between childhood experience and later emotional health (see Ansbacher and Ansbacher, 1956).

The "mental hygiene movement" grew out of the thinking and experience of early American psychologists and mental health workers who provided the stimulus for a movement aimed at guiding parents and educators toward the rearing of children in ways that would strengthen their mental health (see Lamkau, 1956; Levine and Levine, 1970).

Many of these early efforts stressed the importance of recognizing early signs of trouble and taking steps to alleviate the problem or to prevent it from developing into something more significant. Indeed the modern era of primary prevention with children represents a gradual transition from the notion of early intervention with individuals and individual families as a form of prevention to the application of more global approaches to large groups and populations at risk.

The modern developments in primary prevention of emotional distress in children have their origins in the work of many investigators. I will mention only a few pioneers. Skodak and Skeels (see 1949 for summary) did a major series of studies that demonstrated the damaging effect of institutions on children and that have resulted in alternative approaches to the rearing of orphans and foundlings.

Another early influence on efforts to develop a primary prevention orientation was John Bowlby's (1951) book on the role of maternal care and maternal deprivation in infant mental health. His clinical approach was supported dramatically in the series of experimental studies by Harlow (see, for example, Harlow and Harlow, 1966) on the catastrophic effects on infant monkeys (effects that persist into adulthood) resulting from inadequate or non-existent mothering.

Another early innovative program involving an effort at the primary prevention of distress in children was initiated in the 1940s by Loyd Rowland (1969) in Louisiana with his "Pierre the Pelican" series. This series of pamphlets on infant and early childhood care, based on sound mental health principles, was mailed at regular intervals to parents of first born children throughout Louisiana in a program that continues to the present day. The series has been translated into several languages and has been used and evaluated in several cultures around the world.

Another of the pioneers in formulating our concepts and our optimism involving modern primary prevention is Gerald Caplan. He has provided intellectual leadership for more than two decades. In the Winter 1980 issue of the new *Journal of Prevention* Kornberg and Caplan (1980) reviewed the world's literature on preventive efforts with children. In 1955 Caplan edited a book in which the themes emphasizing prevention began to come together as a conceptual model. By 1961 he had edited another book that had a frankly preventive orientation. In the latter book he assembled a number of contributions from people who were immersed in the emerging field of primary prevention with children. Clearly Caplan came to prevention out of a medical orientation that has traditionally emphasized the treatment of the individual. It is interesting to observe him (in his writing) move from an emphasis on the individual child to a concern with the family and the community.

In 1955 he writes:

> Specialists in this field, even though they may be primarily interested in the therapeutic alteration of disordered intrapsychic structure in the child, are working very close in time and in space to the emotional environmental forces whose interplay with the child's developing personality are so important in the etiology of his illness (Caplan, 1955, p. 153).

In 1961 he defines the field as " *'primary prevention'*, i.e., intervention in order to lower the risk of the child's becoming ill with this specific disorder, . . ." (Caplan, 1961, p. 4).

At the same time that the medical orientation of preventing "illness" was gaining advocates, a view that emphasized efforts at "strengthening the host"—positive mental health strategies began to be articulated. Eli Bower wrote a chapter in Caplan's book in which he said: "Primary prevention encompasses actions, deliberative or otherwise, that maximize those social forces in the community which tend to encourage the full development of the human being as a rational, creative, and self-actualizing organism" (Bower, E., 1961, p. 537).

Throughout the 1960s, efforts at primary prevention began to appear in a number of places, including the federal bureaucracy. The Great Society program and the War on Poverty both implied that efforts at prevention could have positive effects on the health, emotional stability, and happiness of children and adults. The program called Head Start is a prime example. (Actually Head Start owes a great deal to a much older program of early intervention with pre-school children started by Maria Montessori, Italy's first woman physician, who devised a whole set of experiences for the children of poverty-stricken families in Trastevere, Rome's worst slum, shortly after the turn of the century.)

By the early 1970s, the idea of primary prevention of child and adult disturbances was taking root everywhere. A first national Conference on Primary Prevention was held at the University of Vermont in 1975 and it attracted a surprisingly large and enthusiastic group of attendees. Their enthusiasm led to the annual conference now established as the Vermont Conference on the Primary Prevention of Psychopathology. Each year the conference papers result in a volume (see Albee and Joffe, 1977; Forgays,

1978; Kent and Rolf, 1979; Bond and Rosen, 1980; Joffe and Albee, 1981; and Bond and Joffe, 1982).

Soon after his election Jimmy Carter established a new President's Commission on Mental Health (PCMH) in fulfillment of a campaign promise. Rosalynn Carter was Honorary Chairperson of the Commission. The Commission established a number of Task Panels to prepare reports on the state of knowledge in various fields of mental health, including a Task Panel on Prevention (1978) which I chaired. Several of the recommendations involving augmented efforts in primary prevention, especially involving special attention to children, were accepted by the Commission and included in their final Report to the President (PCMH, 1978).

There have been three major revolutions in the field of mental health. The first of these occurred when Pinel struck off the chains and brought the insane from the dungeons of Paris up into the light. The humanitarian movement followed. The second revolution was instituted by Freud and led to the gradual understanding of the dynamic causation of mental and emotional disturbances. The third revolution was the development of community based intervention, early help for persons in comprehensive community mental health centers with a variety of services reached through a single entry door.

Now we are on the verge of a *fourth mental health revolution*. It is a revolution involving a shift towards efforts at prevention. It recognizes the impossibility of ever bringing the epidemic of emotional distress under control by attempts at helping single individuals. It accepts the doctrine that prevention is the only meaningful approach to widespread distress.

The fourth revolution makes new demands on those of us already in the field. It means that we must think through our new responsibilities and our new areas of emphasis. We must find ways to untangle the complex web of causation. Practically all discoveries that have led to prevention have been made by our efforts to help individuals, and in the study of their life history. As clinicians we must be alert to the questions of causation and we must encourage our students to be curious about causation.

We must stop focusing our exclusive attention on the individual child, and lift our eyes, shift our focus to the family, the neighborhood, and the community. We must see individual pathology as a reflection of more general social pathology and we must become active in efforts at changing and improving living conditions in our society by reducing needless stress and improving competence and coping skills in children.

We must realize that children of poverty and discrimination constitute a special high-risk group deserving of our attention and help. It is clear that the stress of having an emotionally disturbed or alcoholic father or mother increases substantially the chances of disturbance in the children. We must learn to work with other community agencies in getting help for these high-risk groups.

But most of all, we must change our attitudes toward causation, away from an individualistic and individual pathology model, and toward a more socially-oriented and community-oriented approach to causation and to intervention.

Before this change to a social-causation model can occur, there must be a prior revolution in the thinking of workers committed to helping children and to preventing childhood disturbances. Let us look for a moment at the question of whether we are ready for this revolution.

First of all, for a revolution to begin there must be widespread *injustice*. I suggest that this is the case today. The Report of the President's Commission on Mental Health (1978) identified 32 million persons with serious mental and emotional problems—especially children and adolescents (who were repeatedly identified in the Report as unserved groups). According to the Commission only seven million persons are being seen annually by our mental health system, reflecting a gap that will only get wider and will never be closed. We are neglecting disturbed children and youth, and the elderly, as well as minorities, the rural poor, the urban poor, and the handicapped. So injustice is a condition that widely prevails.

Secondly, a revolution always calls for an *overt challenge to authority*. I believe that the number of voices criticizing medical hegemony in dealing with children's emotional problems has become a large chorus. We are beginning to converge in our theories in the various human service professions that emotionally disturbed children are *not* sick, that the defect model which sees personal taint and genetic or biochemical defect as the causes of all children's mental problems is an invalid model and this insight is leading us to suggest social change rather than medical treatment.

Thirdly, a revolution needs a *clear cut political position* that everyone can understand. The position that I see gaining prominence suggests that "No mass disorder afflicting humankind has ever been eliminated through one-to-one intervention but only as a result of successful prevention." Related to this position in the recognition that *powerlessness* is a major cause of emotional distress, and that the only resolution for powerlessness is a redistribution of power. So the revolutionary political position is that the poor, the minorities, children and youth, women, and other powerless groups must benefit from a redistribution of power.

Fourth, revolutions need a core of *dedicated leaders* with a clear vision of the goals. We have learned a great deal from our brothers and sisters doing one-to-one case work, and psychotherapy. People involved in attempting to help individually distressed and disturbed children and adults have given us a great deal of insight into the social origins of their clients' problems. From these one-to-one interventionists we need to recruit a cadre of leaders who will dedicate themselves to the cause of prevention through redistribution of power.

Fifth, we need to anticipate and be prepared for strong *resistance* from those whose power would be reduced or usurped by our efforts at social change. The medical establishment (including the pharmaceutical industry) is ruthless in its defense of the defect (illness) model. Enormous power and resources are at stake in this struggle. We can expect continued resistance from the mental health establishment to any suggestion that there is not a number of separate and discreet childhood mental illnesses, each with an individual cause, cure, and possible prevention. Our suggestion that human stress results from the injustice and unfairness of the present economic system will result in a powerful counterattack. We already see that funds available for prevention are going to relatively meaningless and trivial projects. It is clear that a great deal of noise will be made about the importance of prevention to cover the fact that little significant work in this area is being supported by the establishment.

Finally, revolutions occur when there is an *unstable power structure*. Again, my reading of the current situation within the helping professions suggests growing instability. Clearly, psychiatry is decreasing in its power and control largely because it is unable to recruit young people into residency training. Twenty years ago when I did a book on the nation's mental health manpower (Albee, 1959) psychiatry was recruiting some nine to ten percent of medical school graduates into its residency programs, and even then the numbers were insufficient to satisfy the need. Recent studies indicate that psychiatry is now recruiting only about 4% of medical school graduates and its popularity continues to decline (Albee, 1979). Only a handful go into child psychiatry. In 1964, when the regulations were written concerning the community mental health centers they stated clearly that every Center had to have a psychiatrist as director. It did not take long to discover that psychiatrists simply were not available for these positions and as a consequence the regulation had to be changed. Today only about one-quarter of all community mental health centers in the country have a psychiatrist as director. Instead, social workers and psychologists have become the responsible administrators.

In short, conditions are ripe for revolution!

But perhaps I am misreading the signs and omens! Back in the days when the world was a much simpler place a great many of us held firmly to the belief that scientific judgments were based on facts, and that social policy changed with accumulating scientific findings, and that theories were held only so long as they were supported by objective evidence.

Those who thought of themselves as politically liberal held to the conviction that the world was slowly and steadily changing for the better and that with improved education, more scientific research, new evidence, and practice eventually society would reach a condition of universal justice and fairness.

I am a slow learner. I no longer believe these things to be true. I now believe that the thirst for power is an addiction, far more dangerous than any other addiction. After reviewing the literature on primary prevention, Marc Kessler and I (1975) said:

> Everywhere we looked, every social research study we examined suggested that major sources of human stress and distress generally involve some form of excessive power. The pollutants of a power-consuming industrial society; the exploitation of the weak by the powerful; the overdependence of the automotive culture on powerful engines—power-consuming symbols of potency; the degradation of the environment with the debris of a comfort-loving impulse-yielding society; the power struggle between the rich consuming nations and the exploited third world; the angry retaliation of the impoverished and the exploited; on a more personal level the exploitation of women by men, of children by adults, of the elderly by a youth-worshipping society—it is enough to suggest the hypothesis that a dramatic reduction and control of power might improve the mental health of people (pp 577-578).

REFERENCES

Albee, G. W. *Mental health manpower trends.* New York: Basic Books, 1959.
Albee, G. W. Psychiatry's human resources: 20 years later. *Hospital and Community Psychiatry,* 1979, *30,* 11, 783-786.
Albee, G. W. The prevention of prevention. *Physician East,* 1979, *4,* 28-30.
Albee, George W. A competency model must replace the defect model. In Bond, Lynne and Rosen, James (Editors). *Competence and coping during adulthood.* Hanover, N.H.: The University Press of New England, 1981.
Albee, G. W. and Joffe, J. M. (Eds.) *The primary prevention of psychopathology: The issues.* Hanover, N.H.: University Press of New England, 1977 (third printing, 1980).
Ansbacher, H. and Ansbacher, R. (Eds.) *The individual psychology of Alfred Adler.* New York: Basic Books, 1957.

Bond, L. and Joffe, J. (Eds.) *Facilitating infant and early childhood experience.* Hanover, N.H.:. University Press of New England, 1982.

Bower, E. Primary prevention in a school setting. In Caplan, G. (Ed.) *Prevention of mental disorders in children.* New York: Basic Books, 1961.

Bowlby, J. *Maternal care and mental health.* Geneva: World Health Organization, 1951.

Caplan, G. (Ed.) *Emotional problems of early childhood.* New York: Basic Books, 1955.

Caplan, G. (Ed.) *Prevention of mental disorders in children.* New York: Basic Books, 1961.

Harlow, H. and Harlow, M. Learning to love. *American Scientist,* 54, 1966.

Joffe, J. M. and Albee, G. W. (Eds.) *Prevention through political action and social change.* Hanover, N.H.: University Press of New England, 1981.

Kent, M. W. and Rolf, J. E. (Eds.) *Primary prevention of Psychopathology: Social Competence in children.* Hanover, N.H.: University Press of New England, 1979 (Second printing 1981).

Kessler, M. and Albee, G. W. Primary Prevention. *Annual Review of Psychology,* 1975, 26, 557-591.

Kornberg, M. S. and Caplan, G. Risk factors and preventive intervention in child psychopathology: A review. *Journal of Prevention,* 1980, *1(2),* 71-133.

Lamb, H. R. and Zusman, J. Primary prevention in perspective. *American Journal of Psychiatry,* 1979, *136,* 12-17.

Lemkau, P. Freud and prophylaxis. *Bulletin of the New York Academy of Medicine, 32,* 1956.

Levine, M. and Levine, L. *A social history of the helping services.* New York: Appleton Century Crofts, 1970.

President's Commission on Mental Health. *Report to the President,* U.S. Government Printing Office, 1978.

Rowland, L. Let's try prevention. In W. Ryan (Ed.) *Distress in the city.* Cleveland: The Press of Case Western Reserve University, 1969. 121-143.

Skodak, M. and Skeels, H. A final follow-up study of 100 adopted children. *Journal of General Psychology, 75,* 1949.

Task Panel on Prevention. President's Commission on Mental Health. *Report on primary prevention.* U.S. Government Printing Office, 1978.

PRIMARY PREVENTION: CHILDREN AND FAMILIES

PRIMARY PREVENTION INTERVENTIONS WITH FAMILIES THAT HAVE YOUNG CHILDREN: THEORY AND PRACTICE

Iris Nahemow, PhD
Genevieve Mann, MS

ABSTRACT. This article describes the theory and practice of preventive mental health programming in one Community Mental Health Center. The Center uses the Albee formula for incidence of maladaptive behavior as a theoretical base. Programming focuses on the denominator factors of problem-solving skills, self-esteem, and support. A description of five types of preventive mental health programs follows the discussion of primary prevention theory.

Introduction

One of the most innovative thrusts of the Community Mental Health Center movement of the 1960's and 70's has been the development of the concepts and practices of primary prevention. Primary prevention in mental health refers to "action taken prior to the onset of mental illness to

Dr. Iris Nahemow is Director of Consultation and Education, Allegheny East MH/MR Center, Inc., Suite 400, Monroeville Medical Arts Building, 2550 Mosside Boulevard, Monroeville, PA 15146. Ms. Genevieve Mann is Supervisor, Early Childhood Team, Allegheny East MH/MR Center, Inc.

intercept its causation or modify its course'' (Goldston, 1977). The term primary prevention, according to Forgays (1978) means lowering the incidence of emotional disorder (1) by reducing stress and (2) by promoting conditions that increase competency and coping skills. This includes improving the quality of life and raising the general level of mental health within our communities.

Dr. George Albee has described primary prevention using the formula below:

$$\text{Incidence} = \frac{\text{Organic Factors} \pm \text{Stress}}{\text{Competence and Coping Skills}}$$

The more balanced the formula, the more likely the individual will be to successfully cope with the stresses in his life. Primary prevention programs therefore aid persons in achieving this balance by providing support, skills, and information, the components in the formulas numerator, in situations where stress or maladaptation are high.

Prevention programs service three groups of people. The first group is persons experiencing normal, developmental crises. These crises are called normal because they occur in most peoples' lives. A normal developmental crisis for a child might be the birth of a sibling or the child starting to school. For adults, examples are marriage, or the birth of a first child. Although these events are common, they are also stressful. They are stressful because they represent changes which require new skills and the leaving behind of old familiar ways.

The second group of people served by prevention programs are those experiencing situational crises such as divorce, death, or a move to a new city. For this group, feelings of loss or fears of helplessness may accompany the stress of solving new problems.

The final group, persons thought to be at high risk for development of emotional disorders, would be those whose life situations would cause greater than usual stress. Examples of this group would be children of emotionally disturbed parents, single teenage mothers, or a child whose parent has died. It is within this group that maladaptation might be most frequently seen.

Those working with children will recognize the situations described above. In fact, many pre-school teachers and day care staff may have an example of each problem area in their current classroom or group. Successful coping with these situations not only allows for the continuation of healthy developmental thrusts, but also contributes to the building of a positive self-image and feelings of confidence around facing future stressful events.

Primary prevention programs may take many forms in actual practice but they usually include the following:

1. Information which provides *anticipatory guidance* (*before* a stressful situation occurs) to enable an individual to better cope.
2. The *support* of caring individuals who have or who now are experiencing the same or similar stresses.
3. *Skills* which can help the individual solve the problems presented by the situation.

A Theory of Primary Prevention Intervention

Allegheny East MH/MR Center, Inc. has provided prevention programs to parents of young children for many years. We have chosen this population as our target group because we believe that the stresses of parenting young children can be brought into balance through this programming. Group attendance is through self-selection, a method which brings together parents of children of an identified age facing similar child rearing issues. The groups are composed of the three types of parents discussed earlier: those experiencing the expected developmental stresses, some experiencing additional situational stress, and some with the more high risk factors. This group composition has been reported by Rose (1974) as giving better results for the more high risk participants, while having no adverse effects on the other participants.

The following program descriptions show how one Community Mental Health Center has attempted to improve mental health and reduce mental illness in its catchment area. We believe that many of our strategies can be used by others who work with children in both pre-school and day care settings, thereby extending the reach of mental health enhancing activities.

Program Descriptions

Early childhood programs are designed for parents and children, newborn through five years of age. Numbers of participants are limited to facilitate discussion among parents and to give individualized attention to children.

The programs are staffed by two child development professionals, one to lead the parent group and the other to be responsible for the children.

Volunteers are recruited and trained to help the staff of the children's groups.

Materials and activities appropriate for each age group are provided by the agency. As the leader of the children's group interacts with the children, she serves as a role model in terms of setting the room environment, and providing the ego support needed to help children grow in competence and self-esteem.

The parent groups focus on developing skills in problem solving techniques and basic communications with children. In addition, parents choose discussion topics such as dealing with stressful situations, sibling rivalry, or building a healthy self-image in children. The parents group leader recognizes the importance of a good self-image in the parent, and models a caring, supportive type of parenting.

Five levels of programming meet the needs of the child participants and their parents. The first of these, *Mother/Infant Programs,* are offered to mothers and babies, newborn to about one year of age, and focus on coping with the changes in lifestyle that occur with the birth of a baby. The program offers support, encouragement, and information about infant development to parents who often feel overwhelmed and isolated in trying to meet the many demands made upon them. Topics for discussion can range from a colicky baby to how Mom can get some needed rest and relaxation. The participants receive anticipatory guidance on upcoming developmental issues and ways to handle specific situations, taking into account their own child's temperament and their unique family situation. This anticipatory guidance helps the parents develop the feelings of competence in problem solving ability.

One indication that this type of program fills the support part of the primary prevention formula is that mothers often express gratitude for a group such as this in which they can receive some nurturing for themselves.

The second program model, *Parent and Junior Toddler Programs,* are designed for the one- to two-year-old and his/her parent. Beginning with this age child, a children's staff provides materials, activities, and facilitation of play while parents meet for discussion at the opposite end of the room. Because these children are at or near rapprochement, every effort is made to allow for the ambivalence of this age child: they may climb up on mother's lap or play independently at the other end of the room.

In the parent's group, issues of separation-individuation as propounded by Mahler (1975) are explored, helping parents understand and cope with the puzzling and frustrating behavior of the now-dependent, now-independent one-and-a-half year old. Oftentimes, the participants have found the group so helpful and supportive, they continue meeting at one another's homes after the formal program has ended.

Next, *Parent and Senior Toddler Programs* go one step further in aiding the separation process for the two- to three-year-old child. The children's group is slightly more removed from the parent's group, being located across the hall or next door. A child may visit with her mother as she feels the need. The children's staff provides a safe and stimulating environment, a variety of activities, and facilitation of play. Major goals are to provide an atmosphere in which children can experience a satisfying relationship to an adult other than a parent, and to learn more about themselves and their peers through play.

Parents of two- to three-year-olds often need extra support, understanding, and suggestions for living creatively with the negative and often out-of-bounds behavior of the toddler. Anticipatory guidance takes the form of exploring methods to prevent situations which encourage negative reactions and power struggles between parent and child. Examining Erik Erikson's (1963) ideas round the two-year-old's needs for autonomy can help parents relax a bit more when topics such as temper tantrums, toileting, and "no-saying" are discussed.

The fourth model, *Parents and Three-Year-Olds,* has children and parents meeting in separate but physically close rooms. Major goals for the children's programs reflect the more balanced, settled disposition of most three-year-olds. Objectives are supporting emotional health (self-esteem, ability to express oneself, the gaining of inner controls, the choosing of one's activities), socialization (awareness of others and their needs, discovering the fun of playing with another, getting what one wants/needs through language development), and opportunities for artistic and creative expression. Through play, we find that children master the developmental issues with which they are dealing at any given time. With the support, encouragement, and modeling of the staff, they can learn problem solving skills which will be valuable to them as they grow.

Parents of these children often want to explore issues such as the effect of a new baby on the three-year-old, handling children's fears and other stressful situations, and how to develop better communications between themselves and their children.

Last, *Parents and Pre-schooler Programs* are often presented in cooperation with school districts for children four to five who will enter kindergarten in the new school year. At times, the programs can be presented in the school in which the children will attend kindergarten, and this can serve as an important transition experience. The focus for the children's group is much the same as for the three-year-old group in terms of goals and objectives around emotional and social growth. The children's leader introduces the children to problem-solving techniques which can be very effective in helping the children learn to communicate meaningfully with one another.

Occasionally, in all five program models, there are parents who feel unusually stressed about their parent/child relationship or about personal problems which cannot be addressed in a group situation. In addition, the staff may recognize the child who is experiencing a difficulty that seems to call for more in-depth intervention. In these cases, appropriate referrals are made in the belief that early intervention can prevent more serious difficulties from arising later.

Summary

The purpose of primary prevention programming is to promote robust mental health in a community, and to reduce the incidence and severity of mental illness. In the Allegheny East catchment area, this is done by providing support, skills training, and anticipatory guidance to parents of children, birth to five-years of age, through the programs described above. The parent evaluations, completed at the end of the programs, indicate that the participants feel we have achieved our objectives. They express gratitude for the realization that they are not alone in the demanding job of parenting. Learning more about child development and being able to share ideas with others are usually high on the list of appreciations.

Our observations of the children at the end of the program sequence show varying levels of growth in competency, problem solving ability, and positive self-image. We also know that most children tell their parents that the groups are fun!

REFERENCES

Erikson, E. H., *Childhood and society,* 2nd ed., New York. W.W. Norton & Company, Inc., 1963.

Forgays, D. G. *Primary Prevention of Psychopathology,* Vol. II. Hanover, New Hampshire: University Press of New England, 1978.

Goldston, S. *Primary Prevention of Psychopathology,* Vol. I. Hanover, New Hampshire: University Press of New England, 1977.

Kane, R. P., M.D., The Family's Role in Primary Prevention. *Journal of Children in Contemporary Society,* 1981, *14*(2/3).

Mahler, M. S., Pine, F. & Bergman, A. *The psychological birth of the human infant; Symbiosis and individuation,* New York: Basic Books, Inc.

Rose, S. D., Group training of parents as behavior modifiers, *Social Work,* 1974, Vol. 19, p. 156-162.

PREPARING CHILDREN FOR SITUATIONAL CRISES

Evelyn Wiszinckas, PhD

A situational crisis is a "dangerous opportunity" to which a child may either succumb through symptom development or other developmental deviation, or from which the child may emerge with increased strength and mastery. Adults can help a child master such stress by the thoughtful preparation of the child for a forthcoming situational crisis. Some guidelines for performing such anticipatory guidance are listed below.

Guidelines For Anticipatory Guidance Work With Children

1. *Preparation of the Adult.* The person who undertakes preventive work with children must recognize the crisis situation as such, become committed to the need for preventive preparation, and then become cognitively and emotionally prepared to do the work. The adult must recognize that any change in the life of a child is stressful. Even events which may be joyous to the adult world, such as the birth of a sibling, will probably involve mixed feelings and require some adjustment on the part of the child. The adult must engage in a supportive dialogue with the child in order to

---

Evelyn Wiszinckas, PhD, was Project Director, Continuing Education Grant, St. Francis General Hospital, Community Mental Health Center, Pittsburgh, PA. She is now Director, Upper Yukon Behavioral Health Service, Fort Yukon, AK 99740.

perceive the significance of such events to the child, then intervene appropriately.

Adults all too often either perceive no purpose in preparing a child for a potentially stressful event, or fear they would unduly alarm the child by doing so. In fact, the danger for the child lies in not engaging in such active preparation. The adult must be committed to the belief that preparatory work is beneficial to the child's optimal development.

The adult must come to some terms with his or her own feelings about the situation in order to most effectively help the child. For instance, a parent's extreme tension about a child's entering school will be communicated to the child in spite of the reassuring words the parent might use. Adults must become aware of their own feelings about the event, consider them, and work with them, either alone or with help, in preparation for working with the child. The adult must also be prepared for experiencing potentially unexpected emotional reactions from the child. For example, whereas a move to a new house may be a happy event for the adults, it may mean the sad loss of favorite things to a child.

2. *Truth.* The child must be told the truth as far as we know it. Keep the truth simple yet accurate. In preparation for an event, the child must be told what is to occur, when, and for how long. The adult need not be concerned about sharing uncertainty with the child. Admit when you don't know something and either seek the answer or share the discomfort of uncertainty with the child. When we keep the truth from children, we leave them at the mercy of their own fantasies. Because of the young child's cognitive and emotional immaturity and lack of experience, the fantasies substituted in place of facts can be quite unusual and often alarming. Such fantasies can be far worse than any reality we can supply. When a child is told the truth, the child can learn to trust.

3. *Repetition and Pacing.* Anticipatory guidance is not accomplished in one sitting. The child needs time to integrate the experience, think of questions, and share varying feelings. At any one time, the child needs to be told only as much as the child needs or wants to know at that time. Major points should be covered first, details may be introduced as needed. A child may need to hear the same thing several times; the child will assimilate at any one time only as much as is manageable. The event should not be the only topic of discussion with the child. The child has other important things to attend to in life. Allow the child to "back away" periodically and return when ready.

4. *Timing.* In preparing a child for an anticipated event (e.g., hospitalization) discussion should begin early enough so that there is time to prepare (not on the way to the hospital) yet not so long in advance that

unnecessary anxiety builds (not a year before the tonsillectomy). Consider the developmental stage of the child; the younger the child, the shorter the time period the child can meaningfully anticipate. Some discussion should begin whenever the family members begin to discuss it among themselves. Family "secrets" and unexplained or unacknowledged upsets can be distressing to a child.

5. *Dialogue.* Anticipatory guidance must be a dialogue, in which a mutual sharing of facts, thoughts, feelings, and questions may occur between child and adult. A lecture given by the adult is not enough. The adult cannot presume to anticipate the thoughts, feelings or fantasies of the particular child; it is only by encouraging the child to share feelings and ask questions that the adult can know what the child needs at that time. The adult must be prepared to alternately lead and also follow the child's lead in the process.

6. *Familiarity.* Unfamiliarity is in itself a stress. When preparing a child for an event, the adult can combat the unfamiliar with real or imagined pre-experience. Let the child know what is to be experienced. When possible, show the child the physical things to be encountered and allow the child to become somewhat familiar with them prior to the event. Encourage exploration of these new things verbally and physically (e.g., hospital equipment, a picture of the new house, a previsit to a new school). If possible, have the child meet the new people to be encountered and, if possible have the child see a trusted adult interacting with them in a comfortable, friendly manner (e.g., the new teacher, doctor, or camp counselor). Many agencies such as hospitals or schools now will not only allow such familiarizing visits but also encourage them. Let the child know what will be expected of him or her (e.g., "it is ok to say ouch") and that the child's basic needs will be met in the new situation (e.g., food, bathroom, sleep, protection).

7. *Feelings.* The child is entitled to whatever feelings he or she experiences related to the situation. In the context of a supportive relationship and in the process of dialogue, the child should be allowed to share these feelings with the adult. The adult cannot presume to always accurately anticipate the extent or quality of the child's emotional reaction to an event. The feelings may be more positive or negative than the adult expects. The adult should keep in mind, however, that some children will frequently laugh as an expression of anxiety. Care must be taken not to misinterpret such laughter. A child's anger is often most difficult for an adult to tolerate, particularly if it is the adult who is responsible for the stressful event (e.g., moving). It is important that the child and the adult learn that their relationship can survive such anger.

The purpose of preventive work is not always to remove the negative feelings associated with the event; the purpose is often to help the child learn to tolerate such feelings (e.g., missing someone).

8. *Anxiety*. Encourage the child's anxiety to be repeatedly mobilized, to a tolerable degree, and acknowledged before offering support. It is difficult for adults to allow or encourage children to be uncomfortable; too often we attempt to remove the stress through assurance and diversion before the child has the opportunity to work with the experience. Through repeated experience with manageable doses of anxiety in a supportive setting, the child's own appropriate coping skills can be mobilized and strengthened for meeting future stress.

9. *Play*. Encourage the child to use play and other favorite modes of self-initiated experience in attempting to master the experience. Children can use imaginative play as a major means of mastering stress. For instance, a child can pretend to be the doctor and administer "shots" to a doll prior to his or her own hospitalization. Other activities which can also be helpful are: making up stories, writing poems, drawing, making up and singing songs. There are many children's books now available concerning potentially stressful events, such as hospitalization, starting school, and moving. These are available at libraries and bookstores. It is important for the adult to know that the preparatory work is not done by the books. Books should be used for information and to stimulate questions and feelings which then should be shared between child and adult.

10. *Support*. Preventive work with the child must be undertaken in an emotionally supportive environment. The major work with the child should be done by those adults who are emotionally closest to the child and with whom the child feels most comfortable. Teachers and other adults who come in contact with the child should be aware of the preparatory work being done so that they can also help. However, the majority of the work should be done by parents and family. There are times when parents, feeling ill-equipped to do such preparation, may ask for help from a teacher or other professionals. It is then important that the professionals' emphasis be on helping the parents do as much of the work with the child as possible, rather than stepping in too readily to do the work themselves. It is also important that all those persons who come into close contact with the child should be in communication with each other so that the work they do is consistent. It is only confusing to a child to be told by a parent that the injection will hurt "like a pinch" only to hear from the physician or nurse "this won't hurt."

Finally, children must be assured that their basic needs will be met, that someone will be available to take care of them, in spite of the uncertainties of the situation.

REFERENCES

Anthony, E. J. *Children at psychiatric risk, Vol. III.* New York: John Wiley and Sons, Inc., 1974.

Bloom, B. L. Prevention of mental disorders: Recent advances in theory and practice. *Community Mental Health Journal.* 1979. Vol. 15(3), Fall.

Furman, E. *A Child's parent dies.* New Haven, Connecticut: Yale University Press, 1978.

Kliman, A. S. Crisis: *Psychological first aid for recovery and growth.* New York: Holt, Rinehart and Winston, 1978.

Kliman, G. *Psychological Emergencies of Childhood.* New York: Grune and Stratton, 1968.

THE FAMILY'S ROLE IN PRIMARY PREVENTION

Ruth P. Kane, MD

ABSTRACT. This article, based on the author's clinical and theoretical knowledge, looks at family intervention in terms of an early intervention primary prevention model. When a family is in some crisis or disequilibrium, the caregiver may intervene in such a way not only to help the family progressively resolve its crisis but also in such a way as to strengthen the family's coping capacities. Anticipatory guidance, strengths, needs, and support are some suggested ways of coping. Developmental aspects of child and family are illustrated by a case example.

Introduction

Much has been written about the varying roles of families in meeting biologic, psychosocial, and sociocultural needs. Particularly in the past generation, both scientific and popular literature has indicated that families often do not promote mental health and in fact are often destructive to the mental health of the family members. Many problems of society, including criminality, juvenile delinquency, child abuse, and schizophrenia have been laid at the feet of the family, most particularly, the mother. Philip Wiley's "Momism," Dr. Ben Spock's alleged permissiveness, the prob-

Ruth P. Kane, MD, is Director of Children and Adolescent Mental Health Services, St. Francis General Hospital Mental Health/Mental Retardation Center, 45 & Penn Avenue, Pittsburgh, PA 15201.

lems of children and youth in the 60's are some examples of this. Within the past two decades, a myriad of literature has been published concerning family therapy, enrolling the family in the treatment of mental and psychophysiologic disorders. A variety of theories have evolved, some of which are interlocking, some diametrically opposed. Very little has been written or discussed about strengthening the family or its potential as a primary mental health promoting institution. The focus of this paper will be to address these issues.

Definition of Primary Prevention

In Sigmund Freud's time, his concept of normality in adults as an ideal to be attained was described as the adult's capacity "zu lieben and zu arbeiten" (to love and to work). I am unaware of a better definition to this day. Prevention has always been an espoused goal of medicine or at least public health. The idea of promoting sound physical health is a familiar one in the public health model. There has been interest in primary prevention since Eric Lindemann's and Gerald Caplan's report on the grief and mourning process following the Coconut Grove disaster in Boston in the 40's. Most of this work in the 50's and 60's has been written by Gerald Caplan or his students. Most recently, psychologists, such as Drs. George Albee, Emery Cowen, and Gaston Blum have also promoted primary prevention. According to classic public health definition, primary prevention consists of those intervention measures aimed at large target populations in order to reduce the *incidence* of mental disorder (rate per 100,000) in a given population. Secondary prevention is defined as concern with those strategies of intervention which will diminish or decrease the *prevalence* of mental disorders or the morbidity factors in a given population by early diagnosis and prompt intervention. Tertiary prevention is described as being aimed at reducing the *deteriorating* effects of chronic mental illness in populations.

Gerald Caplan's description of intervention strategies include several concepts which will be defined. *Crisis intervention,* which is not new with Caplan, but is a concept which he uses in primary prevention, may be defined as those interventions used during a period of disequilibrium or crisis (crisis, in terms of the Chinese symbols means "dangerous opportunity"). A person, group, or system in disequilibrium may exhibit certain tensions and certain qualities of heightened energy which may seek some outlet. Crises are a normative part of life and are either developmental life crises or situational crises. Caplan's notion of crisis intervention involves appropriate, timely intervention at such times which serve to enhance adaptation in a more progressive and/or healthy manner. The alternative to such progressive resolution may be a breakdown of the individual and/or system. In other words, crisis situations may be resolved either progressively or regressively. Appropriate crisis intervention aims at a progressive resolution. *Anticipatory guidance* is a term which describes a process whereby both cognitive and affective information is given before a stressful situation arises, in anticipation of it so that the individual or system may better cope with the situation. Caplan applied *anticipatory guidance* in obstetric clinics in Israel.

George Albee's (1977) definition of primary prevention is expressed in an equation with a numerator and a denominator.

$$\frac{\text{Incidence (New Cases per 100,000)}}{\text{(Mental or Physical Disorder)}} = \frac{\text{Organic} + \text{Stress Factors}}{\text{Competence and} + \text{Self} + \text{Support}\atop \text{Coping Skills} \quad \text{Esteem}}$$

The closer the ratio is to a small fraction, the greater the support, problem solving skills, and competence, relative to the degree of stress and maladaptation, the better prepared is the individual or system to meet stress constructively rather than be destroyed by it.

Cohen-Cole (1978) designed a paradigm which illustrates levels of stress.

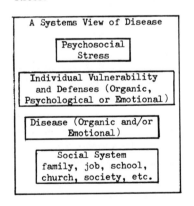

A Systems View of Disease

Psychosocial
Stress

Individual Vulnerability
and Defenses (Organic,
Psychological or Emotional)

Disease (Organic and/or
Emotional)

Social System
family, job, school,
church, society, etc.

Intervention

1. At the level of stress
2. At the level of vulnerability
3. At the level of physiological manipulation
4. At the level of the family

Promoting Primary Prevention in the Family

Just as the individual, for instance the child in the family, grows and develops, it is my contention that families also go through developmental sequences. Perhaps a useful model for looking at development would be to look at the eight stages of man as discussed by Eric Erikson. Bowen's (1976) writings on differentiated families is another model. Families themselves have a developmental course; there is a developmental sequence in their therapeutic process as well. When children are young, families and parents develop along with them, reliving and reworking the past development of parents and other family members. For example, the oedipal-aged child evokes oedipal feelings and conflicts within the family. The latency-aged child may evoke other kinds of issues within family members related to school and learning. Nowhere are the conflicts of the intergenerational problems greater than in the adolescent. In looking at families who present themselves for treatment, one aspect of involvement may be related to where the family is in its own developmental life cycle.

The writings of Mahler, Pine, and Berman (1975) on separation and individuation may be particularly important here in terms of looking at the relative independent functioning of family members as related to the whole. For example, a young father who had not fully differentiated from his family of origin was faced with a dilemma. His eleven month old first born son was protesting when he was left alone by he and his wife. The husband felt the boy was spoiled and instructed his wife to close the door on the boy and leave him alone with his toys. He and his wife could then be together uninterrupted. Since undue separation from his mother represents a developmental trauma to an eleven month old, the intervention given by the Infant Team of the St. Francis General Hospital part F NIMH Primary Prevention Grant was to inform the family of this trauma, give advice and support to the family around other means of sharing parental and husband-wife roles.

Another example was that of an 11-year-old girl who was presented by her parents as having extreme difficulty getting along with her mother. The child had temper tantrums which the mother felt she could not stand. The mother, a very anxious, depressed, emaciated woman, threatened by her illness, wanted to dissolve the family by running away or moving out. The father was extremely threatened by the situation; he supported and was kind to his daughter when the mother wasn't around, yet reinforced the mother's negative, hateful position to his daughter when the mother was there. This example could be looked at in many ways, but one way of looking at the problems is that each family member had great difficulty in separation-individuation. The mother had great difficulty distancing herself from the somewhat hateful, symbiotic relationship that she had with her own alcoholic mother, and saw the 11-year-old daughter as very similar, if not identical, to her mother. The father on the other hand, was driven by a great deal of guilt from many sources. He was an ex-priest, and suffered from many guilts, not the least of which was his guilt about getting married and having children. His wife, and also he, in a more passive way, continued to remain rather dependent on his mother, who is perceived as the "good mother." The 11-year-old daughter, herself, suffered problems during her normative separation-individuation period at age 18 months. The child was sent away during the latter part of mother's pregnancy with a younger brother and remained with the paternal grandparents for several months because mother was ostensibly recovering. The child was very frightened of being sent away and often provoked this feeling. Her behavior was that of a temper-tantrumy, 2½-year-old child; so was that of her mother. The developmental history of course is that of an 11-year-old girl who needs to begin the process of breaking away from her family and the concomitant pre-existing and current conflicts around this developmental crisis.

Certain principles of primary prevention intervention strategies can be applied to the family as a unit as well as to understanding individuals or larger groups in society.

Some primary prevention skills which can be applied to families are as follows: (a) support; (b) education, particularly in problem solving skills interpersonal competence skills; (c) anticipatory guidance; and (d) the strengths-needs approach. For example, family members may need help in supporting one another. This would be helping separation-individuation so that fusion does not prevent the family members from seeing the other person or the situation as identical to theirs, but can be empathetic enough to be supportive in such a way as to help the person to help themselves. In the case of bereavement or grieving in a family where there is a loss, family members should be aware of potential grieving difficulties, particularly those of the children in the family. The perceived loss that children have in relationships is not only that of the lost person, but the loss of the important support provided by that person. Families need to be encouraged to share problems as well as joys.

In the example given before of the 11-year-old girl and her mother, most recently the mother reported that when the youngster returned from another separation from her mother, the mother was able to communicate to the child that she, the mother, was withdrawing from the youngster not because she wasn't glad to see the youngster home, but because she, the mother, was very anxious and scared about how she could handle things and was hoping that she could handle things better but wasn't sure. She also communicated to the child, and this was at nighttime, the separation time, that she thought that perhaps the child, too, was pretty anxious and upset. The child, who had been agitated and upset, was then able to fall off into a peaceful sleep.

Educational approaches which can be used with large groups in society can help the individual family by reducing anxiety, offering alternatives, and increasing problem solving skills. Public media presentations through newspapers, TV, magazine articles, and radio may be utilized to demonstrate principles of mental health. For example, mourning and loss is a part of everyone's life whether there are actual perceived losses or not. The whole process of being born, separated from family, growing up and losing the parent of infancy, the parent losing the young child, are all losses. Other kinds of situational crises, such as death and dying, divorce and separation, moving, and tragedies in the household are also factors which people face. Generally, a crisis point may need to be utilized in order to help families and/or the general public to perceive a need for understanding, consideration, or intervention. For example, in terms of a community disaster, such as flood or holocaust, the anxiety and concern may pull families apart or it may have a potential of pulling them together. Public information about handling stress and utilizing support, particularly of other family members, could be one way to help with the stress problems. Understanding typical reactions to loss may help families cope with stresses or losses by helping them be understanding and by furthering communication within the family.

The competence and problem solving skills probably have been used to a fair degree by family therapists in terms of family oriented tasks and utilizing discussion for alternative means of problem solving. It is my contention, however, that many family therapists use a somewhat directive approach which may solve the individual problem and solve it quite well, but may not go on to promote families' interpersonal problem solving skills.

Anticipatory guidance utilized in groups also helps in terms of promoting curative factors within groups. Through this approach there is support; there is knowledge that there are other people in the same boat and that there will be anxiety but that nothing is so terrible that it may not be discussed or talked about.

Anticipatory guidance in terms of work done with the Part F NIMH Grant, with which I am associated, includes prenatal parent support groups both in clinics and with private patients. Parents are led in anticipating labor and delivery, as well as the oncoming anxieties associated with them. They are also led to anticipate some of the probable concerns and problems both in the marital relationship and in the extended family and with the child himself.

Other *anticipatory guidance* activities have been utilized in Well Baby Clinics in terms of helping parents know what to expect with the oncoming developmental stages of children, discipline problems, etc. *Anticipatory guidance* could also be utilized in helping members anticipate the family's entrance into a new developmental stage. Even if the family is seen for a specific problem, once the problem is solved, some discussion about what may happen in the future may be done using a variety of techniques, such as role playing, family sculpting, or mere discussion.

There is research evidence to support the potential efficacy of intervention strategies, such as anticipatory guidance. Broussard and Hartner (1976), have conducted longitudinal studies on normal first born neonates. Broussard's assumptions that the maternal perception of her normal neonate at one month of age is predictive preventive ingredients. The importance of early condition, right start, etc., has a predictive value for adjustment later in life, as seen in parent-child relationships, husband-wife relationships, education, job attitudes, and success. Appropriate self-esteem building by *anticipatory guidance* has been studied by the St. Francis General Hospital Mental Health Center's Part F NIMH Grant in Primary Prevention and Early Intervention for "at risk" children 0–8 years and their caregivers. Expectant parent support and education groups which offer opportunities for active mastery have shown positive results in the mother's labor and delivery experience—especially clinic patients as documented by hospital and physician records. A preliminary study on Prenatal Prediction of Psychosocial Risk for Children has been developed by Part F NIMH Grant Staff. Maternal perception of her post delivery supports and her relationship with her own mother have been found to be predictive of subsequent development of her child. Negative maternal prenatal perceptions may well be altered by anticipatory guidance and support, not only of the expectant mother, but also her family—husband, boyfriend, and parents (the latter two particularly with unwed mothers and teenagers). School adjustment by system and individual child intervention has been another facet for primary prevention. By offering support and informational problem solving groups to teachers in preschool and kindergarten through third grade, a child's adjustment—his separation and individuation from family—is enhanced.

The strengths-needs approach also may be applied to families. Certain families may enjoy a certain amount of masochistic gratification in complaining and seeing how negative and terrible everything is. Some family interactions are based almost entirely on problems and negative expectations. The role of the family therapist or group leader in providing a different model for identification may be seen. For example, looking at strengths in a family may be something quite foreign to the family. Caught up in their own day-to-day problems and being distraught, the family may not be able to look at and utilize their strengths, or may minimize them, being continually fixed on negativism and problems. Although a therapist may encounter considerable initial resistance in emphasizing strengths, such an approach may help the family to find and use its inherent strengths. Working with agency caregivers in perceiving the needs and strengths of their clients may be helpful in terms of preventive family system intervention. Working with, for example, "at risk" children in families, working with medical caregivers, social service workers, and educators in a consultative educative way may help these caregivers perceive their clients in different more positive ways.

Implications For Future Family Therapy

With the additional focus of primary prevention, a family therapist can recognize the importance of preventing future problems. The family therapist can go one step beyond treating specific ills and can strengthen the family's ability to cope with future problems, thus preventing future illness or at least decreasing its intensity. Perhaps we can really utilize the notion that an ounce of prevention is worth a pound of cure.

REFERENCES

Albee, G. *Primary Prevention of Psychopathology,* Vol. 1. Hanover, New Hampshire: University Press of New England, 1977.
Bowen, M. Family therapy, theory and practice, *Theory and Practice of Psychotherapy.* New York: Gardner Press, Inc., 1976.
Broussard, E. R. and Hartner, M. S. S., MD, Maternal perception of the neonate as related to development. *Child Psychiatry and Human Development,* 1976, 7(2).
Caplan, G. *Prevention of Mental Disorders in Children,* New York: Basic Books, Inc., 1961.
Cohen-Cole, S. A. MD, Depression. *Medical Digest,* Inc. 1978.
Mahler, M., Pine, F., & Bergman, A., The psychological birth of the human infant. New York: Basic Books, Inc., 1975.

LEARNING TO WALK
IN A BRAVE NEW WORLD:
PREVENTION AND INTERVENTION WITH
INFANTS AND FAMILIES

Robin F. Woods, PhD

ABSTRACT. A primary concern of prevention is the infant "at risk" for a variety of disorders. The area of greatest concern is the area of human attachment. Attachment is a process of developing a relationship with a significant other. Signs of the existence and quality of an attachment include use of the significant other for: (a) familiarization, (b) gratification of needs, (c) comfort, (d) affectivity, and (e) as a secure base from which to explore. Using the new body of knowledge about man's infancy, it is possible to develop prevention programs that follow a five step process: (1) setting goals and objectives; (2) screening and identifying a population; (3) assessment of strengths and needs; (4) selecting appropriate intervention methods; and (5) evaluation.

A primary concern of the sphere of "Prevention" during the past few years has been the infant "at risk." "At risk" is a term widely used and seldom defined. In any meeting of prevention professionals, a number of those in attendance will identify themselves as working with infants "at risk." When asked, "At risk" for what?, the answer will often be, "At

Robin F. Woods, PhD, is a Research Consultant for the Parental Stress Center of Pittsburgh and Child Development Specialist for the Penn Group Health Plan, Pittsburgh, PA 15206.

risk'' in the area of development. The next question is, ''Which area of development?'' The answer to that question is usually sufficiently confused as to be a non-answer. It is not unusual to hear, ''at risk for a wide variety of disorders,'' and then to find that there are no terms to list in the ''variety.'' This world of prevention with ''at risk'' infants is a Brave New World where as yet few ''honest'' answers have been defined. It is a world where tentative steps have been taken, and where directions are still being sought.

A thorough understanding of man's early years is a body of knowledge still in its infancy. Yet several things have become clear. One of these areas of clarity is that man's psychobiosocial nature is readily observed in the human infant. The human baby does not develop first physically, then socially, then psychologically, but rather develops as a whole *system,* all aspects of his/her person developing simultaneously and uniquely. All aspects of the human being also develop in interaction with each other and in interaction with the environment.

Each baby is born with a set of inheritances—his or her unique history—for no human being is without a history. This history is made up of inheritances—the psychobiosocial inheritances and genetic factors from both father and mother, and the basic characteristics of being human. As a human, man is a social animal, designed in total psychobiological structure to establish relationships with other human beings. A normal, healthy baby is ready at birth to use his human sensory-response capacities to begin interacting with the people in his environment.

It is this ability of such tiny, dependent creatures as human babies to reach out and participate in the development of a relationship with another human being that has become a fundamental concern of prevention with ''at risk'' infants. Of special concern is the relationship of mother and infant—the infant-mother system. The infant-mother system established during pregnancy and the immediate post-partum period—the first six weeks of a baby's life—is seen as being a particularly significant time in terms of ''later outcome.'' The ''later outcome'' concept is generally implied as being a ''developmental outcome.'' There is still much confusion about what is needed by ''at risk'' infants, what can be done about what is needed, and how to tell if what was done was effective.

Gradually, some things have become clear. While ''at risk'' may refer to a variety of circumstances, most often the ''at risk'' mother-infant system is seen as being ''at risk'' in the area of *attachment.* Attachment is the term used to describe the existence of a relationship between mother and child. The early work of René Spitz (1965) established that a meaningful relationship was necessary in order for a baby to survive. Even a tiny infant needs to matter to someone. What is being examined now is the *quality* of the infant-mother attachment, not simply the presence or absence of a relationship.

An attachment is a relationship. As a relationship, attachment is interactional in nature. Human attachment has been identified as vital to the developing child (Bowlby, 1969). Bowlby (1969) called attachment a normal human process that takes place between mother and child during the first year of life. Ainsworth and Bell (1973) defined attachment as an affectional tie one person forms between himself and another specific one, a tie that binds them together in time and space and endures over time. As an affectional tie and as a process, attachment receives a contribution from both the mother and the child (Bell, 1974, Brazelton, 1974). An attachment means the presence of reciprocity of systems; this reciprocity involves affects—emotions, and means that there is a qualitative aspect to the process of attachment.

Attachment might also be called love. It is more than an affect. Attachment is made up of interactions of all the affect from joy to contempt. Izard (1977) has called love an affective-cognitive structure—a bond, tie, or strong association with an image, word, thought, or idea. To the infant, mother ultimately becomes all of these things—an image, a mental representation, a word—*mother,* a thought—a memory of an experience, or an idea—anticipation of an experience. To the mother, *infant* is ultimately all these things as well. This affective-cognitive structure is a process of a particular child becoming the child of a particular mother, a process Margaret Mahler called the *Separation-Individuation* process (1975). As an affective-cognitive experience of two particular individuals, the attachment process involves feelings that are demonstrated through observable behaviors. The infant who singles out the mother for preferential smiling and begins to cry at the sight of stranger (Spitz, 1965) is demonstrating attachment behavior. An important characteristic of attachment behavior is that it is discriminatory in nature (Bowlby, 1969. Ainsworth and Witig, 1969), and that it tends to evoke a response from the object of attachment "which initiates a chain of interactions which serves to consolidate the relationship" (Ainsworth, 1964, p. 50).

Attachment between mother and child is the beginning relationship on which all other relationships depend. Within the field of infancy there has been a growing consensus that this initial *attachment* is a training ground for all other relationships, and that if other psychosocial functioning is going to be optimal and appropriate as a person grows, this infant-mother relationship needs to be as positive as possible. Enter then, the first, tentative steps of preventive intervention, a first hypothesis: Do as much as possible to facilitate optimal attachments, and many disorders of a psychosocial nature will be prevented.

Around the world, programs have begun to explore this first hypothesis. There are many approaches to this exploration. Some programs are short, some are indefinite in length. Some deal only with parents, using parent education as a method; some deal primarily with the babies, attempting to give the babies a "corrective emotional experience." Some deal with the total family system. Each is hoping to find new horizons that will help not only children and families, but also the explorers who want to help children and families.

There are many specific programs that could be reviewed in depth, and many that are becoming fundamental in the literature—a new body of knowledge about a new demension of human development. The intervention programs under the direction of Stanley Greenspan at NIMH, Elsie Broussard in Pittsburgh, Pennsylvania, and Selman Fraiberg at the University of Michigan are just three of the projects that have produced exciting discoveries related to methods of intervention. The pioneering work of Betty Tableman and the Office of Prevention within the Michigan Department of Mental Health has led to some new understandings of program goals, objectives, and outcomes. The Michigan Infant Mental Health Association has been a prime mover in encouraging the development of community programs to promote optimal development of infants and their families.

A close look at the results of these various efforts reveals that there is a five step process that can facilitate the designing of prevention programs for infants and families. These steps are: (1) establishing goals and objectives; (2) screening and identifying a population; (3) assessing the strengths and needs of the population to be served; (4) selecting the techniques of intervention; and (5) evaluating the program. These are the first steps of this Brave New World.

The setting of clear goals and objectives is essential to an intervention or prevention project; if the other steps are to follow adequately, goals must be clearly stated. The goal of a project may be to lower the incidence of child abuse or psychiatric disorder by facilitating the optimal development of mother-infant attachment. The methods of intervention will be designed to address objectives toward achieving this goal.

Identifying the population most in need of a preventive intervention service requires finding a method of screening the population. A frequent problem faced by programs is finding an adequate method of screening. There are some screening instruments that identify infants that may be "at risk" in the area of attachment. The Broussard Neonatal Perception Inventories (1979) screen on the basis of maternal perception. The Michigan Office of Prevention has developed an instrument that utilizes a variety of factors, including observation of mother-infant interaction during the immediate post-partum period (1979). The important thing is that the instrument being used, or screening method being used is designed to identify infants at risk in the area of human attachment, whatever the circumstance that places them "at risk."

Screening serves to identify a population which may have a significant proportion of infants in distress in the area of attachment. The next step is to do a careful clinical assessment of the population identified to further clarify the nature of that population. The nature of intervention is that it builds on strengths, as well as attempts to overcome weakness. Assessment must generally be done on a case by case, individual basis, using individual interviews and clinical observation of mother-infant interaction. A body of knowledge has been emerging during the last decade that indicates a general consensus regarding specific areas of assessment of significance in the area of attachment. These include: (a) use of mother for familiarization, (b) use of mother to gratify needs, (c) use of mother for comfort, (d) use of mother for affective expression (pleasure to unpleasure), (e) use of mother as a secure base. These areas are some of the areas that need to be included in a clinical assessment within a program that wishes to intervene in the area of human attachment.

Once a population has been screened and assessed, intervention is ready to begin. There are many types of intervention—individual, group, educational or interactional, short term or long term. Some models that have been used "successfully" with a variety of populations include: *Anticipatory Guidance, Parent Education, Support Groups, Home Visitations,* and *External Services.*

Anticipatory Guidance models are generally designed to be used with large populations where an in-depth clinical assessment is not part of the program. Anticipatory guidance models provide parents with information about problems they or their infants may encounter as they get to know each other. An underlying philosophy of *anticipatory guidance* is that if parents anticipate that some problems may occur, they will be better able to cope with whatever problems may happen.

Parent Education models are usually designed to give specific solutions to specific problems. These models include concrete information about normal child development and alternative, appropriate ways parents can respond to children. There is usually a clearly designed curriculum with materials each parent may purchase.

Support Groups can take a variety of forms. Many times these groups are organized around a strong group leader who consciously attempts to provide a parenting role to participants in the group. The model is often referred to as "mothering the mother." The *support group model* is not designed around a rigid curriculum, but rather takes its cues from the group members. Group members are encouraged to learn from each other, and to share their successes and accomplishments as well as their anxieties and fears. Support groups may run for short, contractual periods, or for long periods, with termination times being determined by the group participants.

Home Visitation models are an intensive, almost therapeutic model, utilizing a single home visitor who visits the family on a regular basis, usually weekly or bi-weekly. Frequently, intervention of this type is utilized when the screening and assessment process has identified an infant/family system in extreme distress. The home visitation model is particularly useful when a family is actually or psychologically isolated.

Another method of intervention is done by providing families with necessary *External Services*. This may include transportation to clinics and doctors appointments, delivery of needed household items and other services which may be unique to a given family. In these models, which may sometimes be combined with other models, no therapeutic interaction is attempted. Services are provided with the hope that a family will appreciate being cared for, and that this knowledge will then be transferred to family interactions.

All of these types of preventive intervention are being used with mother-infant systems where concern about attachment and the quality of mother-child interactions is the focus of the program. The type of intervention should be selected according to program goals, screening findings, and the results of the clinical assessment.

Evaluating such programs has been a challenge that is difficult to meet. Evaluation procedures must be designed to fit the initial screening and assessment procedures as well as the ongoing assessment procedures that are an integral part of any intervention method. Even with screening and assessment, how do you know you have prevented something? The absence of the undesirable phenomenon is the primary criteria for proving that a project has accomplished its goals.

Some of the first attempts at evaluation of projects designed to have an impact on the infant's capacity for affective relationships utilized developmental scales and indices. However, these measures, such as the Bayley Scales of Infant Development, assess areas of cognitive and psychological functioning rather than areas of social relationships, and do not have areas for evaluating mother-infant attachment. Attention is now being paid to evaluation procedures designed to assess mother-infant interactions and the affective functioning of the infant. The Infant Mental Health Profile (Woods, 1979) and the Greenspan and Lieberman (1980) procedures regarding contingent and anti-contingent behaviors are examples of measures designed to assess attachment and affectivity.

And so, there does appear to be a rhythm and design, a logic, around the new world of "prevention" with the infant "at risk." In the winter of 1974, Selma Fraiberg addressed a standing room only crowd in the auditorium of Western Psychiatric Institute in Pittsburgh, Pennsylvania. Mrs. Fraiberg described a fledgling undertaking begun at the University of Michigan Child Development Project. The Infant Mental Health movement had begun. Infant Mental Health is still a new field. Many discoveries have been made and many hypotheses formed during the ensuing seven years. It is a firm hypothesis that many known psychosocial disorders have their roots in the earliest human experience. These have been just the first steps into a new world. That new world—that Brave New World—of what may someday be seen as Attachment Therapy—is only one dimensional at this point. It is like a world of surface images—there is a shape, but its place in time and space is not yet known. These dimensions have yet to be explored. The direction for new explorations can be taken from the experience of those pioneers who have been establishing new and exciting programs for "at risk" infants and their families.

REFERENCES

Ainsworth, M.D. Patterns of attachment behavior shown by the infant in interaction with his mother. *Merril Palmer Quarterly, 1964, 10,* 51-58.

Ainsworth, M.D., & Bell, S. M. Attachment, exploration and separation: Illustrated by the behavior of one-year-olds in a strange situation. *Child Development,* 1973, 49-67.

Ainsworth, M.D., and Wittig, B.A. Attachment and exploratory behavior of one-year-olds in a strange situation. In B.M. Foss (Ed.), *Determinants of infant behavior IV.* London: Methiven, 1969.

Bell, R.I. Contributions of Human Infants to Caregiving and Social Interaction. In M. Lewis, & L.A. Rosenblum. *The Effect of the Infant On the Caregiver.* New York: John Wiley & Sons, 1974.

Bowlby, J: *Attachment and loss: Attachment.* New York: Basic Books, 1969.

Brazelton, T. B. Early parent-infant reciprocity. In M. Lewis, & L.A. Rosenblum. The effect of the infant on the caregiver. New York: John Wiley & Sons, (Eds.), 1974.

Broussard, E.R. Assessment of the adaptive potential of the mother-infant system: The neonatal perception inventories. *Seminars in Perinatology,* Vol 3, No. 1 (January) 1979.

Greenspan, S.I. & Lieberman, A.F. Infants, mothers, and their interaction: A quantitative

clinical approach to developmental assessment. Available through authors, Center for Clinical Infant Studies, National Institute of Mental Health, Bethesda, Maryland.
Izard, C: *Human Emotions.* New York: Plenum Press, 1977.
Mahler, M: *The Psychological Birth of the Human Infant.* New York: Basic Books, 1975.
Spitz, R. *The first year of life.* New York: International Universities Press, Inc., 1965.
Tableman, B. Office of Prevention, State Department of Mental Health, Lansing, Michigan.
Woods, R.F. The Infant Mental Health Profile. Pittsburgh, Pa. 1979. (Available through the editor of this issue).

DEVELOPING COPING SKILLS
IN EARLY CHILDHOOD:
THEORY AND TECHNIQUES

Sandra L. Forquer, PhD

ABSTRACT. Techniques for fostering the development of coping skills in early childhood are proposed in this paper. The differences between pseudo-immunity to stressful events vs. psychological immunity are highlighted. Emphasis is placed on the role of the community caregiver in facilitating the development of problem-solving skills in preschool populations. The introduction at new challenges in manageable dosages is highly encouraged.

Growing Up Isn't Easy

"Growing up isn't easy" has served as a proverbial sign post for describing the process of passing through the normal developmental tasks between infancy and adulthood. Issues of trust vs. mistrust, autonomy vs. prolonged dependency, feelings of omnipotence vs. recognition of vulnerability in toddlerhood, and the separation anxiety that accompanies preschool entry make up a set of normal, predictable developmental tasks that a youngster strives to master during early childhood.

Sandra L. Forquer, PhD, is Director of Primary Prevention, Systems Research Unit, Eastern Pennsylvania Psychiatric Institute, Henry Avenue and Abbottsford Road, Philadelphia, PA 19129.

Fostering successful mastery of these normal developmental tasks has become the focus of study in recent years (Anthony, 1973; Murphy and Moriarity, 1976). Anthony has observed both children at low risk and high risk for the development of mental disturbances. At-risk factors are defined as "givens" in either the physiological or psychological environment of the child, i.e., poor housing, malnutrition, congenital defects, family discord, parental mental illness. In addition to assessing the risk factors present in a given situation, Anthony contends one must also assess the level of vulnerability of the child. Vulnerability refers to the child's ability to withstand and successfully cope with both a stressful environment and the stress that is inherent in accomplishing normal developmental tasks. A child can be at high risk for developing a disorder because of physical, environmental, and socio-economic factors. Yet, that same child can also possess a high level of invulnerability to those risk factors due to psychological preparedness and the presence of support systems.

The fostering of psychological preparedness to withstand risk factors and successfully master developmental tasks is inherent in the concept of developing coping skills in early childhood. Community caregivers, i.e., day care staff, nursery school staff, and pediatric nurse practitioners can play vital roles in fostering the development of coping skills in a preschool population.

Mastery: From Where Does It Sprout?

Anthony has defined mastery as a force generated in the individual that leads him to test his strength against his environment and to assert himself. For example, the transition from standing up to walking requires numerous trials and errors before the joy of mastery of that developmental task can emerge. Opportunities for autonomy need to be provided. "Benign neglect" vs. overprotectiveness creates a healthy environment for exploration and mastery. In describing the vulnerable personality, Anthony borrows from mythology, conjuring up the image of Achilles. As we recall, Achilles' mother afforded him a type of "fake" protective shield by plunging Achilles into the river Styx at birth. By so doing, his whole body was rendered "invulnerable" except for his heel from which she had held him. Yet, his mothers' attempts to provide immunity failed dismally. Achilles' heel was vulnerable; he had been provided either with a pseudo-invulnerability.

Contrast Achilles' experience with that of Hercules. In the case of Hercules, he was continuously exposed to a series of problems which required him to utilize his own initiative, strength, and problem-solving abilities. Hercules strangled a lion, conquered the Cretan Bull, recovered the golden apple. As Hercules successfully completed each task, his problem-solving abilities expanded and he felt competent about his own abilities to master his environment. Hercules was truly the mythological character developing a type of psychological immunity to stress and risk factors. That "immunity" involved an internal, active process vs. the external, passive type of immunity provided Achilles.

The roots of mastery then, are part of a process learned very early in life of how one interacts with one's environment.

Coping Styles of Preschoolers

Murphy and Moriarity wanted to know what coping patterns normal children utilized. They defined coping as a general term to include active ways of handling stress and solving problems. Inherent in their definition is an assumption that the struggle will meet with at least some success. In their study of children in Kansas, they observed both the child's ability to cope with opportunities, challenges, frustrations, and threats in their environment as well as his/her ability to maintain his own internal organization and functioning. In other words, was the style of coping with stress relatively free from marked stress, unmanageable anxiety, loss of motor coordination?

At the preschool level, any deterioration or inhibition of cognitive motor or integrative function was viewed as an indication of vulnerability. Extreme physical or affective reactions to stimulation were viewed similarly.

Coping styles observed in the preschoolers in their study included:

1. Temporary regression: thumbsucking, foot-tapping, lip play.
2. Strategic withdrawal: ability to fend off excessive stimulation by taking a "rest."
3. Ability to select from or restructure the environment, i.e., change activity or actively work to solve problem.
4. "Freezing" or tightening up of muscles.
5. Fuzzy speech, stammering or speech distortions.
6. Loss of motor coordination.
7. Uncontrollable emotional outbursts, clinging.

Techniques for Developing Coping Skills in Early Childhood

The community caregiver who is involved with the preschool population can be quite facilitative in encouraging the developing of coping skills that will contribute to a sense of competence and self-esteem. Either through direct contacts with the children or through indirect contacts with the parents of this age group, the community caregiver can serve as an educator, a facilitator and most important, a source of ongoing and available support.

Two complimentary approaches to developing coping skills and fostering a sense of competence will be presented here. The first approach focuses on maintaining the internal integration of the child by teaching the child to recognize and utilize his own resources. This approach additionally introduces manageable new challenges into the environment. These challenges are aimed at building psychological immunity and preparedness for dealing successfully with stressful events. The second approach is the didactic teaching of problem-solving techniques to preschoolers. This latter technique, developed by Spivack and Shure (1978), involves the use of dialogue as a means of facilitating cognitive interpersonal skills.

A. Approach I Techniques

1. Observing child and record coping styles (utilize list in preceding section).
2. Allow for temporary regression as a protection against vulnerability.
3. Facilitate resilience by timing rests, encouraging withdrawals, recommending changing activities.
4. Communicate with the child about what you are doing. Alert him/her to his/her own cues, encourage insight, recommend a constructive coping style as a means of helping the child manage his/her vulnerability.
5. Recall that vulnerabilities are not static; as the child develops more resources for coping with stress, the susceptability to particular stressors will change. Depending on the developmental task to be mastered, there will be periods of higher vulnerability as compared to periods of lowered vulnerability.
6. Be prepared to introduce new challenges in manageable doses in order to facilitate the child's ability to cope successfully with stress.
7. Create an environment that provides strong support coupled with "benign neglect." By thus permitting and encouraging exploratory and curiosity behaviors, the child will be encouraged to test his abilities to master new tasks.

B. Approach II Techniques

The work of Spivack and Shure has demonstrated that it is beneficial to teach nursery-school children the ICPS approach (Interpersonal Cognitive

Problem-Solving). They have identified a set of variables that have had a significant impact on adjustment. In this approach children are taught that they have within themselves the availability of resources for problem-solving. Preschoolers are taught alternate-solution thinking followed by consequential thinking:

Problem: Johnny grabbed the red truck from me and I want it back.

Alternate-Solution Thinking: (a) I could grab it back; (b) he could have the green one; (c) we could take turns.

Consequential Thinking For: (a) I might lose; (b) he'll say no; (c) we can both use it sometimes.

The Spivack and Shure approach to teaching cognitive skills has been packaged and includes teaching aids, scripts for training parents on how to teach problem-solving techniques to their children.

Summary

The techniques enumerated above are intended to foster the development of coping skills in early childhood. The role of the community caregiver in this process is emphasized. Two mythological characters were introduced to depict the difference between providing a pseudo-immunity to stressful events vs. providing an immunity based on the child's knowledge of his own resources, coping styles, and problem-solving skills. The continuing introduction of new challenges in manageable dosages is highly encouraged as a means of building both competence and self-esteem. It is furthermore emphasized that life involves a series of normal, predictable, developmental tasks that are accompanied with joy when mastery is achieved. Growing up isn't easy, but we do possess the know-how to facilitate the development of coping skills that can contribute to better social adjustment and positive outcomes to stressful situations.

REFERENCES

Anthony, E.J., *Children at psychiatric risk.* New York: John Wiley & Sons, Inc. 1974.

Kliman, G. *Psychological emergencies of childhood.* New York: Grune & Stratton; 1968.

Murphy, L.B., & Moriarity, A. *Vulnerability, coping and growth.* New Haven: Yale University Press, 1976.

Shure, M.B., & Spivack, G. *Problem-solving techniques in childrearing.* San Francisco: Jossey-Bass Publishers, 1978.

COMMUNITY SUPPORT SYSTEMS
AND THE NEIGHBORHOOD:
A PROSE POEM WITH NARRATIVE

Phillip Pappas, MEd

ABSTRACT. Issues and causes rise and fade in the American awareness with an incredible intensity and swiftness. As our focus is directed to the next "crisis" we allow ourselves to believe that yesterday's problems have been resolved. Acutely aware that this is not the case, a group of concerned people from the professions, government, and residents without any special training of any sort, began to meet regularly in 1970 to see in what ways the quality of life in the inner city might be improved.

Out of these meetings came the understanding that control of the services required for the maintenance and growth of neighborhood life is an essential precondition for personal and family growth. Furthermore, the will to achieve this control is derived from the strength of the bridges built between neighbors.

Those of us involved with
neighborhood support systems
over the years
have grown weary
always concerned with what
categorical funds, what stream

Phillip Pappas, MEd, is Director of the Community Human Services, 374 Lawn Street, Pittsburgh, PA 15213.

what title speaks to
neighbors supporting neighbors

But recently as if by some magic
the dialogue in mental health
has coined new concepts
networking
support systems
of course with caution
an exclusive focus on target populations
• the chronically mentally ill
• children
all of which translates back to
the street
neighbors
neighborhoods

The problem facing neighborhoods, families and their children is the lack of discretionary funds, funds without categories that permit the neighborhood, through its natural networks, to develop systems of care controlled and operated by the neighborhood. Our success in South Oakland in Pittsburgh, an integrated neighborhood of 5,000 people, stems from the courage exhibited by Allegheny County Mental Health and Mental Retardation to allocate funds for the project without imposing arbitrary guidelines. These funds provided a small group of us with the opportunity to settle in the neighborhood, to open up a storefront, and to listen.

The action finally comes back
to the stoop (the porch)
where on a summer day
neighbors talk, react to
the screaming parents
the abused child
the lady with the long dress
and funny smell
the abandoned but proud elderly
the beer hidden under the bed
"talking about themselves"
all the behavior
the gossip

the concern
and care
originates here
and extends
naturally
neighbor to neighbor

Listening and inviting neighbors to informal activities are the first ingredients of a needs assessment, a capacity to understand the strengths and
weaknesses of the neighborhood. Through bingo, an open classroom for
children, a cadre of neighbors organized with a primary focus on socialization, on celebration, on sharing food. This cadre began to develop trust
with us, with each other. Over time, some six months the cadre on its own
initiative conducted street by street meetings. The purpose was to talk,
share and explore the needs of the neighborhood. The process was natural,
unassuming, . . . and without setting expectations, an assessment was
made of neighborhood needs.

—Two-parent families dissolving at a record rate.
—Psychological depression in an unsteady economy.
—Expanded role of women with inadequate supports for child rearing
and health maintenance.
—Youth alienation, drug culture, and crime.
—A position on elderly which cuts them from their family ties, where
the nourishment that age, wisdom, cultural and ethnic backgrounds can
offer to the young, is allowed to atrophy and vegetate.
—Lack of primary health care facilities.

It is this energy, these concerns
that need marshalled
organized

in the form of *governance*
how do we govern our destiny
how do we restore ourselves
our neighborhoods

which leads to the question
of *competency* and action
how do we help
what skills do we need

who can teach us
who can help us care for
our troubled
and ill

The key words are governance and competence. How do we organize ourselves to address these needs? Since we, neighbors, identified the issues, how do we establish the priorities with an emphasis on neighborhood control of the system of care? Given the 60's and the O.E.O. movement the notion of governance became closely linked with the political system. It was not uncommon for the ward leader to develop a Board of Directors reflecting his or her interests and to establish a service system for the neighborhood that was an extension of patronage. In our experience, however, the neighbors asked for open nominations, open elections, which they conducted by knocking on each door in the neighborhood. Over ninety people were nominated and election was held in key areas in the neighborhood. Under these conditions the ward leader lost handily to a Polish lady who had no political experience but who in time became a moving force in the neighborhood. The Board, which got elected, reflected all the ethnic, racial, and class interests of the neighborhood. Although such a Board leads to extensive meetings, arguments on priorities, pressures on the workers in the care system, it becomes the first step towards control. Governance is the crucial element needed in developing a neighborhood support system.

From governance, it is natural to move toward development of a system of care. It is important however, to raise the second question— competence. By competence we must not presume that once the needs are identified, and a governance model established, the system of care must be delivered by professionals. It is imperative at this stage that the neighborhood, through its leadership, identify neighbors who have skills, who can be trained, who care, to become front line, the providers of the service. Again this takes time and begins with informal programming. Since socialization was an important need and this led initially to bingo games, dances, parties at Christmas, it was natural for neighbors to plan and organize these events. Food became an important ingredient and one which related to the neighborhoods competency. (Pierogies were more important than advocacy.) Given this competency, a cadre of women moved from planning bingo games and ethnic fairs to developing, within three years, a nutrition program that now feeds 130 people daily. Building on this success, neighbors became concerned about the health needs of the elderly, the chronically mentally ill, and the children. At the same time, they requested some planning and training from health assistants. They were especially interested in providing health care in peoples homes. Over three years the Health Assistant Program became a comprehensive primary care health system serving over twenty five percent of the population. Again, a movement from informal care models to a nurse oriented health care station staffed by nurse practitioners and doctors. It was clear at this junction, after some five years, that continuity of care became a crucial issue focused again on the elderly, chronically mentally ill, and children. It is uncommon for a neighborhood to solicit funds for a group home. But, since this was a recognized need, the neighborhood planned and implemented a home for the elderly and chronically mentally ill, again staffed by them and connected to the nutrition and health care systems. This increased focus on continuity of care led naturally to programs for children and families. Beginning informally with a mothers day out, the neighborhood grew to provide a pre-school, kindergarten, and a day care program for over sixty children. This concern with child rearing led to a parents association and a single parents group that has extended its concerns to the public school which led to a neighborhood-run language arts center in the local school. Plans are now underway to extend day care into peoples homes, hopefully increasing the opportunities for families that must work to survive. All of this, of course, costs money and there is some dependence on public funds. But since these programs have been organized and operated by neighbors a fee structure was developed. Even though the neighborhood is poor, the neighborhood raises thirty percent of the cost to operate all the programs.

When neighbors organize, control, and deliver systems of care they not only serve specific populations in need but also create those informal networks that extend the care system to all in the neighborhood. Their concerns mushroom into self-help networks for the elderly, single parents, and youth with an emphasis on integration of classes and races. When the neighborhood ran a summer day care program in the woods, it was attended by infants, mothers and fathers, youth, elderly, and chronically mentally ill. It is these informal care networks that extend the formal programming and become the ingredients for neighborhood preservation and growth.

But as stated earlier, this takes time—in our case some ten years. Although the system depends almost exclusively on neighbors providing the service, becoming the front line, the role of the professional is still important.

The source of our malaise
as professionals
is
that we have forsaken
forgotten
buried
the stoop in all of us
its trauma
its nurturing
we have grown away from it

But we are still children
nurtured in support systems
sometimes negative
sometimes positive
remember
running in the streets
fighting our wars
dreaming of becoming
doctors
firemen
husbands
wives
John Wayne
Greta Garbo
saviors of the world
heros and heroines
but fully grown
and somehow abstracted
somehow trained
somehow cynical

We are afraid to return
because at first blush
we cannot protect ourselves
we cannot use our skills
or show our house
or our new car

But hopefully if we take the risk
we can rediscover the
stoop in each of us
and help our neighbors and ourselves

The professional can be a magician or an anathema to many who see their role principally as providers of service. We would argue, however, that the needs and the problems are too great, too comprehensive, and too intimately connected with a neighborhood life style for the professional to have significant impact. Instead we must become brokers, trainers, negotiators for the neighborhood. We must provide, sometimes magically, the occasions for neighbors developing systems of care governed and delivered by them. We must provide the opportunities for dreaming, for shaping vision. It is only then that neighbors will understand that some of the problems, some of the issues can only be handled by trained counselors, surgeons, therapists, architects, and accountants.

Given these concerns
this dreaming
neighborhood support systems
re/emerge

The re/emergence
often needs the gadfly
the modern shaman

who help people, neighbors
recall their roots

the stoop (porch) is in all of us
we have been networked
we have been supported

in me it has been the culture
of music and dance
celebration, laced with guilt

a pagan/christian sense
of extending
outward to embrace
to help
sometimes gracefully
often awkwardly

but remembering always
the stoop
and stripping the intellectual baggage
of degrees, skills
that makes the stoop

an edifice
an institution
a treatment mode
a labeling of pain
a labeling of class and race
this does not suggest that we don't
need the baggage

But we do need the balance
between the kid
who left the stoop
to become a professional
a businessman
a therapist

the possibility of rediscovering
the stoop in each of us
and returning to our roots
and the
simple
but complex concern of neighbors
struggling to defy
the steady diet
of anonymity
boredom on the job
lack of intimacy
lack of money
bitter todays and tomorrows

PRIMARY PREVENTION: CHILDREN AND THE SCHOOLS

Emory L. Cowen, PhD

ABSTRACT. First, a working concept of primary prevention is presented and the need for greater emphasis on such programming is developed. Children are seen as logical prime targets for primary prevention program efforts and schools are considered to be natural sites for such programming. Examples are given of ongoing work in: (a) early detection and intervention, (b) programs based on the helper-therapy principle, (c) mental health education, (d) competence training, (e) social system analysis and modification, and (f) stress reduction and coping with stress, each an area thought to hold special potential for future primary prevention work with young children in schools.

For centuries—indeed, since its inception—the mental health field has steered a fixed course. Just as physicians are society's designated caregivers for the body and its ailments, mental health's charge has been to comprehend and restore "sick minds."

Notwithstanding that fixity of heading mental health is considered to have passed through several revolutions each of which significantly modified how society defined and dealt with psychological problems (Zax & Cowen, 1976; Rappaport, 1977). The first, engineered by Phillipe Pinel in

Emory L. Cowen, PhD, is Professor of Psychology, The University of Rochester, Rochester, NY. This article was written with the partial support of a grant from the NIMH Experimental and Special Training Branch (MH 14547-04). The author acknowledges that support with gratitude. Requests for reprints can be mailed to the author, The University of Rochester, Department of Psychology, Rochester, NY 14627.

the late 18th century, aimed at sweeping humanitarian reform in the care and treatment of the profoundly ill. Freud was father to a second revolution that vastly expanded mental health's scope—i.e., its view of the nature, causes, and treatment of psychic dysfunction. Although that revolution brought a new hope and optimism, today, nearly a century after it started, we realize that it has neither resolved mental health's ancient, refractory problems nor new ones identified as the field's purview broadened. Thus two major clusters of failings of the mental health system remain in plain view: (1) Limited resources are directed first to crystallized adverse "end-state" conditions (e.g., psychoses, neuroses, character problems)—deeply-rooted psychological problems that most resist change. (2) Scarce resources are packaged and distributed in ways that are not accessible to large segments of society—often those who most need help.

Growing awareness of those vexing problems has created ferment and a clearer recognition that mental health's past ways are insufficient to today's problems. *Bonafide* new alternatives are needed. One such set, i.e., the recent community mental health (CMH) thrust, protests against the narrowness and ineffectuality of past approaches. At its core, it is an active, systematic search for better ways to bring effective services to many more people, including particularly the heretofore unreachable (President's Commission Report, 1978). Powered by that goal, the movement has been operationalized by significant developments in early detection and screening and active outreaching interventions built on that base, mental health consultation, crisis intervention, and the use of new atraditional help-agents in an effort to cope with diverse psychological problems.

Although the contributions of the CMH movement have been significant and "liberalizing," they have not overcome many of the problems identified as the scenario of the second revolution unfolded. In the final analysis, CMH less challenges the gut assumptions or directions of past mental health approaches (i.e., to diagnose and treat dysfunction) than it does to raise serious questions about whether established practices are the only or best ways to implement those assumptions.

The omnipresent specter of weighty, unresolved mental health problems serves as a continuing prod to explore fresh, effective, socially utilitarian solutions. In that spirit, a qualitatively different family of alternatives is now gestating that goes well beyond mere challenges to past mental health practice to raise questions about its pivotal assumptions. Just as public health (preventive) medicine recognized that no disorder could be overcome by treating its victims (Bloom, 1979) and that certain heretofore baffling conditions could be prevented, so are we coming to recognize that it may be more sensible, pragmatic, humane, and cost-effective to build health from the start and to prevent dysfunction than to struggle, however skillfully and compassionately, to minimize its costly, devastating residuals.

That is the essential kernel of primary prevention, built on a view long-known to successful military generals and football coaches, i.e., a good offense is the best defense. Primary prevention has several key defining or marker-qualities. It is mass-oriented to groups before the fact of maladaptation. Although primary prevention programs can be targeted to those "at risk," engaging already-established maladjustment in individuals is beyond its territorial limits. Primary prevention is also "intentional," i.e., its programs strive either to build health and competencies in people from the start or to prevent adverse psychological outcomes. In other words, it seeks to bring about felicitous outcomes by: (a) judicious application of educational approaches; (b) the constructive modification of systems, settings and environments; (c) reducing sources of stress and training people to cope more effectively with stress; and (d) promoting psychological health. It thus calls for different skills and techniques than those used by mental health in the past.

The Prevention Task Panel of the President's Commission on Mental Health (1978) argued appropriately that young children are ideal targets for primary prevention programs:

> Primary prevention's defining characteristics and mandates necessarily structure its main strategies. With proaction, health and competence-building, and a population-quality among its core qualities, it follows, virtually automatically, that primary prevention programs must be heavily oriented to the very young. (p. 1840)

If young children are, indeed, ideal targets for primary prevention programs, the lion's share of such work must, for several reasons, be done in schools. First, children spend great portions of their waking hours in school during their formative years (Bardon, 1968). Second, schools, more than any other social institution, provide convenient access to large numbers of children. And third, education is both the natural vehicle for, and backbone of, primary prevention programming. In other words, there is a natural symbiosis among primary prevention programming, young children, and the schools.

Primary prevention can be done in many different ways (Cowen, 1980). Moreover, lines of demarcation among primary, and other forms of prevention (e.g., ontogenetically early secondary prevention) are often blurred. Thus, some programs include both primary and secondary prevention components and others with an initial secondary prevention thrust move in primary directions as they evolve.

The rest of this paper describes several types of "pure" primary prevention programs, and programs with significant primary prevention components, for young school children.

1. *The Primary Mental Health Project (PMHP),* a program for systematic early detection and prevention of school adjustment problems, has been in operation for 24 years (Cowen, Trost, Lorion, Dorr, Izzo, Isaacson, 1975). It, and several conceptually related programs such as the St. Louis County Mental Health Project (Gildea, 1959; Gildea, Glidewell & Kantor, 1967; Glidewell, Gildea & Kaufman, 1973; Rae-Grant & Stringer, 1969) and the South San Francisco PACE ID program (Brownbridge & Van Vleet, 1969) share the goals of: (a.) systematic early screening of young children to identify youngsters "at-risk" and (b.) providing prompt effective helping services to such children to prevent later more serious problems. PMHP's active help-agents are nonprofessional "child-aides," i.e., housewives, carefully selected for their warmth, effective interpersonal relationships, and skills and comfort in working with young children (Cowen, Dorr & Pokracki, 1972). The professional role-model in PMHP is that of a mental-health "quarterback" who recruits, trains, and supervises an expanded cadre of child-aides and is a resource person and consultant for other school personnel. That revamped delivery mode dramatically expands services to large numbers of children-in-need (Cowen, Lorion, Kraus & Dorr, 1974). Moreover a series of PMHP outcome studies (Cowen et al., 1975) demonstrates that the intervention is highly effective. Recently, PMHP has been involved in active program dissemination (Cowen, Davidson & Gesten, 1980) leading to the adoption of the model by more than 300 schools in 50+ school districts around the country.

Although PMHP began as a program in ontogenetically early secondary prevention it later developed true primary prevention components. Two small examples: (a) Consultation, an important element in PMHP, often deals with class management problems that teachers are having with children. As teachers acquire knowledge in that sphere and apply it effectively to new classroom situations, they are taking important steps toward primary prevention. (b) One PMHP research study (Felner, Stolberg, & Cowen, 1975) showed that children who experience life- and family-crises such as parent separation, divorce, and life-threatening illness or death in the family, have more serious school adjustment problems than demographically matched referred peers who have not experienced such crises. Based on that finding, PMHP developed a short-term intervention for youngsters experiencing current life crises, but not yet showing maladaptive symptoms (Felner, Norton, Cowen & Farber, 1981). Such a before-the-fact intervention, when effective, exemplifies true primary prevention. More directly, PMHP has used its successful secondary prevention program as an entree for developing true primary preventive programs based on competence training and modification of the social environment of primary grade classrooms (cf. below).

2. *"Helper-therapy" principle.* Some years back, Riessman (1967) developed an innovative program to meet the mental health needs of the urban poor. Using accessible neighborhood store-fronts as service delivery bases and disenfranchised inner-city workers as service-providers, he found both that the services were helpful to "consumers" and that the help-agents grew *personally* through the process of helping distressed others. The latter occurrence is the quintessential element of the helper-therapy principle. The principle is entirely consistent with Staub's (1979) later conclusion, based on a review of empirical studies with children, that successful participation in live helping interactions with others is among the most important factors in shaping a child's prosocial behavior. The gut notion behind Riessman's and Staub's conclusions, based on different perspectives, circumstances, data-bases, and age groups is that people help themselves when they provide meaningful help to others. Properly harnessed the principle holds much potential both for prevention and for developing mutually enhancing resolutions of complex social and human adaptive problems, including those facing young school children. School based programs that can incorporate the helper-therapy concept include those in peer-teaching, coaching, and the creation of mutual support groups.

Effective applications of the helper-therapy principle in school settings illustrate how prevention objectives—primary, for the help-agent, and early secondary, for the young school-age target child—can be met through a single, carefully engineered program. Illustratively, Cowen, Leibowitz, and Leibowitz (1968) described a program in which retired people worked effectively as help-agents with early maladapting primary grade school and Tefft (1975) reported a similar program in which tuned-out junior high and high school students filled comparable roles with primary graders experiencing school adjustment problems. Both programs resulted in twinned gains, i.e., for help-agents and helpees.

3. *Education,* rather than diagnosis and treatment, is a key gateway to primary prevention with children. A variety of educational approaches—cognitive and affective, direct and indirect—have been explored with that goal in mind. An early example is Ojemann's (1961, 1969) work in "causal education," an approach that teaches causes, analytic processes,

and understandings in contrast to typical "surface" approaches that seek to impart facts. Behind the causal education model is the assumption that a child who acquires analytic skills and competencies will be able to cope more effectively with adaptive demands, i.e., to adjust better. Support for that assumption comes from evaluations of several causal training programs with 4th–6th graders, demonstrating such outcomes as reduced anxiety and insecurity, growth in self-concept, improved peer sociometric status, and more positive overall adjustment profiles (Bruce, 1958; Muuss, 1960; Griggs & Bonney, 1970). In a related vein, Baskin and Hess (1980) reviewing the effectiveness of seven different types of affective education programs (e.g., Teacher Education Training (TET); Developing Understanding of Self and Others (DUSO)), concluded that such programs result in gain in cognitive, overt behavioral and internal-emotional functioning particularly the first two.

Some educational programs with primary prevention goals are indirectly targeted, e.g., parents are the direct participants, though the program's goal is to improve *children's* adjustment. Thus following a parent education program conducted by Hereford (1963) the *children* of parent participants improved significantly in relationships with classmates even though they themselves were not part of the program. A program for low-income Mexican-American families combined home and family education with an actual nursery school experience for young children (Johnson & Breckenridge, 1981). That program led to improved parent-child interaction patterns in participant families and direct adjustment gains, e.g., less hostility and greater considerateness, in program children. Heber's (1978) comprehensive educational program for the (at-risk) children of intellectually limited mothers illustrates the same generic approach to prevention programming.

4. *Competence Training.* In contrast to the preceding, broad-gauge, educational approaches to primary prevention, other educational programs with comparable goals teach *specific* competencies or families of competencies that are thought to mediate positive adjustment. For example, based on a long line of prior research demonstrating that maladjusted or clinical groups, at various age and SES-levels, are deficient in a cluster of interpersonal cognitive problem solving (ICPS) skills such as alternative solution, consequential, and means-end-thinking (Spivack, Platt & Shure, 1976), programs have been established to train young children in such skills (Spivack & Shure, 1974; Allen, Chinsky, Larcen, Lochman & Selinger, 1976; Gesten, Flores de Apodaca, Rains, Weissberg & Cowen, 1979). The primary prevention potential of that work resides in the possibility that ICPS skill acquisition mediates behavioral adjustment. Evidence

is now available to suggest that children do, indeed, acquire ICPS skills through training and that, as that happens, their adjustment improves (Spivack & Shure, 1974).

Although ICPS skill training is currently the most popular in the family of competence-building approaches to primary prevention (Urbain & Kendall, 1980), it is not the only such approach. Anderson and Messick (1974) describe 29 different social competencies in young children, many of which may have important relationships to adjustment. Some therefore are appropriate targets around which to build primary prevention programs. Examples of competence training programs in other areas can be cited: Stamps (1975) taught realistic "goal-setting" to inner-city 4th grade children, and demonstrated that successful acquisition of those skills was accompanied by improvements on personality and behavioral measures. Susskind (1969) and Gall (1971) have conceptualized curiosity and question-asking behaviors in young children as competencies that can facilitate learning and adaptation. Although the content of the preceding areas differ, each represents a teachable skill for which curriculum can be developed and which can be taught to as yet unaffected groups of children to upgrade specific competencies and to help them to adapt more effectively.

Other competence training programs reported in the literature fall in the gray area between primary and early secondary prevention because they are targeted to children who may already be manifesting *some* early difficulties. Illustratively, La Greca and Santagrossi (1980) report an effective behaviorally oriented training program for children evidencing early social skill deficiencies. The program, which teaches children specific skills such as joining groups, sharing, cooperating, and engaging in conversation led to improved role-playing skills and a greater ability to initiate peer interactions. Related approaches for children with early social skill deficiencies have been developed by Oden and Asher (1977) and Oden (1980) who use "coaching" techniques for such youngsters, and by Hartup and his associates (Hartup, 1979; Furman, Rahe & Hartup, 1979) who paired socially inept children with 18 months-younger, socially normal children, as a way of strengthening the former's social skills. O'Connor (1972) has compared the efficacy of several approaches such as shaping and modeling for reducing the negative effects of social withdrawal in young children.

Because the competence approach is mass-oriented, before-the-fact, and based on educational technology, it offers an attractive paradigm for future primary prevention work in the schools (Prevention Task Panel Report, 1978). At the broadest level, its key questions are: Which core competencies or skills mediate adjustment? Can curricula and training models be developed to impart those skills to young children? Can it be shown, empirically, that when that happens adjustment also improves? (Cowen, 1977).

5. *Social system analysis and modification* is yet another attractive approach for primary prevention work. High impact social environments such as those of the family and school significantly shape young children's psychological development for better or worse. They are, in other words, anything but neutral in their effects. The ultimate challenge that that reality poses is how to engineer environments, e.g., the social environment of primary grade classrooms, to optimize young children's educational and personal development. That question implicates a complex, three-stage process. A first requirement is to develop sensitive measures of class environment. People such as Moos (1979) and Stallings (1975) have already made significant contributions to that area. Once such measures are available the next need is to chart relationships between environment properties and relevant educational and personal outcomes. For example, Trickett and Moos (1974) found that student satisfaction was high in classes seen as high in involvement and as having close teacher-student relationships. Other recent studies have shown that elementary classes seen as high in order and organization, involvement and affiliation, compared to their opposite numbers, have students with more positive mood states, greater peer acceptance, and higher teacher-rated adjustment (Wright, 1980), as well as better self-control (Humphrey, 1981). As environment-outcome relationships are established, the major challenge for primary prevention is to use such information effectively to engineer class environments that optimize educational and personal outcomes in children. An example of that approach is the work by Aronson et al. (1978) on "jig-saw" classrooms. In jig-saw teaching, children work together on projects in small groups. They must rely heavily on each other to piece individual findings into a cohesive communal report. Cognitive gain is one outcome of that process; another, with special relevance for primary prevention, is that it fosters better morale, improved self-esteem, and warmer, closer interpersonal relationships among children (Aronson et al., 1978). Other steps toward engineering the environment of classrooms to promote children's adaptation and well-being are reported by Moos (1979).

6. *Stress reduction and coping with stress.* Consistent relationships have been shown between stress and life crises on the one side, and psychopathology and maladaptation on the other (Dohrenwend & Dohrenwend, 1974; Dooley & Catalano, 1980). Crisis situations have been described as times of both danger and opportunity. Ineffectually handled they leave lasting psychological scars; well-handled they can strengthen the

person's future coping abilities (Caplan, 1964). A case in point: Each year thousands of young children experience new, threatening, medical, surgical, and/or dental procedures. Because such experiences are anxiety-producing, they are often followed by serious short-term, or long-term, emotional difficulties. An emerging body of data suggests that, through the use of expressive and modeling procedures, children can learn to cope effectively with such crises (Melamed & Siegel, 1975). Graziano, De-Giovanni & Garcia (1979) summarize that work and cite its implications:

> . . . modeling may be an effective aide in preparing children for dental and medical treatment, thus reducing their possibly high situational fears . . . In all of these studies the strategy was a preventive one, i.e., prior to the occurrence of the stressful situation children were prepared so that they could more effectively cope with stress when it did occur. There are important implications for prevention and stress innoculation approaches. (p. 818)

The last sentence of the above quote warrants emphasis. It is part of the very fabric of childhood that children will, sooner or later, experience stressful life events. For some, the very fact of school entry is stressful. For others, painful medical/dental procedures, the birth of a sibling, separation or divorce of parents, or life-threatening illness or death of a close family member may be stress-precipitants (Felner et al., 1975). Children are highly vulnerable at such times. Accepting that reality and building effective programming around it can surely advance school-based, primary prevention efforts with young children.

Primary prevention approaches offer the mental health field a clear, attractive set of alternatives. Because such approaches seek to prevent difficulties before they happen and to build competencies in people from the start, education is their natural vehicle. Hence, schools represent the most sensible sites for such efforts and young, flexible, modifiable children their most obvious targets. Examples have been cited of promising primary prevention program-directions with young children in schools. A concerted effort to develop programs of that type would surely help to redress serious imbalances in current delivery systems and, thus, ultimately to resolve some of mental health's chronically vexing problems.

REFERENCES

Allen, G. J., Chinsky, J. M., Larcen, S. W., Lochman, J. E., & Selinger, H. V. *Community psychology and the schools: A behaviorally oriented multi-level preventive approach.* Hillsdale, N. J.: Lawrence Erlbaum Associates, 1976.

Anderson, S., & Messick, S. Social competence in young children. *Developmental Psychology*, 1974, *10*, 282–293.

Aronson, E., Blaney, N., Stephan, C., Sikes, J., & Snapp, M. *The jigsaw classroom*. Beverly Hills, Ca.: Sage Publications, 1978.

Bardon, J. I. School psychology and school psychologists. *American Psychologist*, 1968, *23*, 187–194.

Baskin, E. J. & Hess, R. D. Does affective education work? A review of seven programs. *Journal of School Psychology*, 1980, *18*, 40–50.

Bloom, B. L. Prevention of mental disorders: Recent advances in theory and practice. *Community Mental Health Journal*, 1979, *15*, 179–191.

Brownbridge, R., & Van Vleet, P. (Eds.). *Investments in prevention: The prevention of learning and behavior problems in young children*. San Francisco, Calif.: Pace ID Center, 1969.

Bruce, P. Relationship of self-acceptance to other variables with sixth-grade children oriented in self-understanding. *Journal of Educational Psychology*, 1958, *49*, 229–238.

Caplan, G. *Principles of preventive psychiatry*. New York: Basic Books, 1964.

Cowen, E. L. Baby-steps toward primary prevention. *American Journal of Community Psychology*, 1977, *5*, 1–22.

Cowen, E. L. The wooing of primary prevention. *American Journal of Community Psychology*, 1980, *8*, 258–284.

Cowen, E. L., Davidson, E., & Gesten, E. L. Program dissemination and the modification of delivery practices in school mental health. *Professional Psychology*, 1980, *11*, 36–47.

Cowen, E. L., Dorr, D., & Pokracki, F. Selection of nonprofessional child-aides for a school mental health project. *Community Mental Health Journal*, 1972, *8*, 220–226.

Cowen, E. L., Leibowitz, E., & Leibowitz, G. The utilization of retired people as mental health aides in the schools. *American Journal of Orthopsychiatry*, 1968, *38*, 900–909.

Cowen, E. L., Lorion, R. P., Kraus, R. M., & Dorr, D. Geometric expansion of helping resources. *Journal of School Psychology*, 1974, *12*, 288–295.

Cowen, E. L., Trost, M. A., Lorion, R. P., Dorr, D., Izzo, L. D., & Isaacson, R. V. *New ways in school mental health: Early detection and prevention of school maladaptation*. New York: Human Sciences Press, Inc., 1975.

Dohrenwend, B. S., & Dohrenwend, B. P. *Stressful life events: Their nature and effects*. New York: Wiley, 1974.

Dooley, D., & Catalano, R. Economic change as a cause of psychological disorder. *Psychological Bulletin*, 1980, *87*, 450–468.

Felner, R. D., Norton, P. L., Cowen, E. L., & Farber, S. S. A prevention program for children experiencing life crisis. *Professional Psychology*, 1981, *12*, 446–452.

Felner, R. D., Stolberg, A. L., & Cowen, E. L. Crisis events and school mental health referral patterns of young children. *Journal of Consulting and Clinical Psychology*, 1975, *43*, 305–310.

Furman, W., Rahe, D., & Hartup, W. W. Social rehabilitation of low interactive preschool children by peer intervention. *Child Development*, 1979, *50*, 915–922.

Gall, M. The use of questions in teaching. *Review of Educational Research*, 1971, *40*, 707–721.

Gesten, E. L., Flores de Apodaca, R., Rains, M. H., Weissberg, R. P., & Cowen, E. L. Promoting peer related social competence in young children. In M. W. Kent & J. E. Rolf (Eds.), *The primary prevention of psychopathology, Vol. III: Social competence in children*. Hanover, N. H.: University Press of New England, 1979.

Gildea, M. C.-L. *Community mental health*. Springfield, Ill.: Thomas, 1959.

Gildea, M. C.-L., Glidewell, J. C., & Kantor, M. B. The St. Louis school mental health project: History and evaluation. In E. L. Cowen, E. A. Gardner, & M. Zax (Eds.), *Emergent approaches to mental health problems*. New York: Appleton-Century-Crofts, 1967.

Glidewell, J. C., Gildea, M. C.-L., & Kaufman, M. K. The preventive and therapeutic effects of two school mental health programs. *American Journal of Community Psychology*, 1973, *1*, 295-329.

Graziano, A. M., DeGiovanni, I. S., & Garcia, K. A. Behavioral treatment of children's fears: A review. *Psychological Bulletin*, 1979, *86*, 804-830.

Griggs, J. W., & Bonney, M. E. Relationship between "causal" orientation and acceptance of others, "self-ideal self" congruence, and mental health changes for fourth- and fifth-grade children. *Journal of Educational Research*, 1970, *63*, 471-477.

Hartup, W. W. Peer relations and the growth of social competence. In M. W. Kent & J. E. Rolf (Eds.), *Primary prevention of psychopathology, Volume III: Social competence in children*. Hanover, N. H.: University Press of New England, 1979.

Heber, F. R. Sociocultural mental retardation: A longitudinal study. In D. G. Forgays (Ed.), *Primary prevention of psychopathology, Volume II: Environmental influence*. Hanover, N. H.: University Press of New England, 1978.

Hereford, C. F. *Changing parental attitudes through group discussion*. Austin: University of Texas Press, 1963.

Humphrey, L. L. Relationships between class environment variables and children's self-control. Unpublished Ph.D. Dissertation, University of Rochester, 1981.

Johnson, D. L., & Breckenridge, J. N. Primary prevention and the Parent Child Development Center. Paper presented at APA Meeting, Toronto, Canada, 1978.

La Greca, A. M., & Santagrossi, D. A. Social skills training with elementary school students: A behavioral group approach. *Journal of Consulting and Clinical Psychology*, 1980, *48*, 220-227.

Melamed, B. G., & Siegel, L. J. Reduction of anxiety on children facing hospitalization and surgery, by use of filmed modeling. *Journal of Consulting and Clinical Psychology*, 1975, *43*, 511-521.

Moos, R. H. *Evaluating educational environments*. San Francisco, Ca.: Jossey-Bass, 1979.

Muuss, R. E. The effects of a one and two year causal learning program. *Journal of Personality*, 1960, *28*, 479-491.

O'Connor, R. D. The relative efficacy of modeling, shaping and the combined procedure for the modification of social withdrawal. *Journal of Abnormal Psychology*, 1972, *79*, 327-334.

Oden, S. L. A child's social isolation: Origins, prevention, intervention. In G. Cartledge & J. F. Milburn (Eds.), *Teaching social skills to children*. New York: Pergamon, 1980.

Oden, S. L., & Asher, S. R. Coaching low-accepted children in social skills: A follow-up sociometric assessment. *Child Development*, 1977, *48*, 496-506.

Ojemann, R. H. Investigations on the effects of teacher understanding and appreciation of behavior dynamics. In G. Caplan (Ed.), *Prevention of mental disorders in children*. New York: Basic Books, 1961.

Ojemann, R. H. Incorporating psychological concepts in the school curriculum. In H. P. Clarizio (Ed.), *Mental health and the educative process*. Chicago: Rand-McNally, 1969.

Prevention Task Panel Report, *Task Panel reports submitted to the President's Commission on Mental Health, Vol. 4*. Washington, D. C.: U. S. Government Printing Office, Stock No. 040-000-00393-2, 1978.

Rae-Grant, Q., & Stringer, L. A. Mental health programs in school. In M. F. Shore & F. V. Mannino (Eds.), *Mental health and the community: Problems, programs and strategies*. New York: Behavioral Publications, 1969.

Rappaport, J. *Community psychology: Values, research, and action*. New York: Holt, Rinehart & Winston, 1977.

Riessman, F. The "helper" therapy principle. *Social Work*, 1965, *10*, 27-32.

Riessman, F. A neighborhood-based mental health approach. In E. L. Cowen, E. A. Gardner, & M. Zax (Eds.), *Emergent approaches to mental health problems*. New York: Appleton-Century-Crofts, 1967.

Spivack, G., Platt, J. J., & Shure, M. B. *The problem solving approach to adjustment*. San Francisco, Ca.: Jossey-Bass, 1976.

Spivack, G., & Shure, M. B. *Social adjustment of young children*. San Francisco, Ca.: Jossey-Bass, 1974.

Stallings, J. Implementation and child effects of teaching practices on Follow-through classrooms. *Monographs of the Society for Research on Child Development*, 1975, *40*, (Serial No. 163).

Stamps, L. W. *Enhancing success in school for deprived children by teaching realistic goal setting*. Paper presented at Society for Research in Child Development, Denver, 1975.

Staub, E. *Positive social behavior and morality (Vol. 2): Socialization and development*. New York: Academic Press, 1979.

Susskind, E. Encouraging teachers to encourage children's curiosity: A pivotal competence. *Journal of Clinical Child Psychology*, 1979, *8*, 101–106.

Tefft, B. Underachieving high school students as mental health aides with maladapting primary grade children: The effect of a helper-helpee relationship on behavior, sociometric status and self concept. Unpublished doctoral dissertation, University of Rochester, 1975.

Trickett, E. J., & Moos, R. H. Personal correlates of contrasting environments: Student satisfaction in high school classrooms. *American Journal of Community Psychology*, 1974, *2*, 1–12.

Urbain, E. S., & Kendall, P. C. Review of social-cognitive problem solving interactions with children. *Psychological Bulletin*, 1980, *88*, 109–143.

Wright, S. Perceived environment and its relation to student outcome. Unpublished Ph.D. Dissertation, University of Rochester, 1980.

Zax, M., & Cowen, E. L. *Abnormal psychology: Changing conceptions, 2nd Ed*. New York: Holt, Rinehart & Winston, 1976.

PLANNING PRIMARY PREVENTION PROGRAMS: A PRACTICAL MODEL

Sandra L. Forquer, PhD

ABSTRACT. This paper proposes a model for primary prevention activity planning. It provides the practitioner with a framework for identifying multiple variables affecting a population, a means for assessing which variables to address and a structured approach to planning preventive interventions.

The limitations of the model appear to be current limitations of the field. The technology for weighting risk factors and stressors, the quantification and weighting of skills and supports is under development.

Introduction

As the 1978 Report to the President from the Mental Health Commission has indicated, the incidence of mental disorder in the United States continues to rise. Increases in the incidence of mental disorders are associated with societal signs of economic recession and high unemployment. However, these economic events also reduce the availability of

Sandra L. Forquer, PhD, is Director of Primary Prevention, Systems Research Unit, Eastern Pennsylvania Psychiatric Institute, Henry Avenue and Abbottsford Road, Philadelphia, PA 19129. This is an abridged version of a paper presented at the Primary Prevention Symposium sponsored by the Smoky Mountain Mental Health Center, Dillsboro, North Carolina, October 13–17, 1980. The full text will be published in a monograph of the conference proceedings early in 1982.

funds for provision of services to populations in need. As financial resources dwindle, new approaches to analyzing service delivery arise in
response. The 1980's have been heralded in with recurring cries for
"cost-effectiveness," "time-limited services," and more "efficient"
utilization of resources. The entire field of human services must answer
critical survival questions about whom they serve, for what purpose, and at
what cost.

Human service practitioners are themselves under stress as the realities
of scarce resources lead to job reductions and higher levels of job expectations for a smaller number of personnel. Staff feel overburdened, under-
payed, and often "burned out." The one-to-one therapeutic approach fails
to reduce the line at the door; in fact, with the reduction of job slots, the
line can indeed become longer, contributing to the practitioners' sense of
futility (Albee, 1978).

Primary prevention offers practitioners an opportunity to promote mental health and to keep the "mentally healthy" healthy. It affords the practitioner an opportunity to make use of knowledge accumulated over time
about general and specific populations and about the risks and stresses
which people experience as part of everyday living. Prevention provides
the practitioner with the means of building competency and coping skills in
individuals, groups, or communities toward the planned outcome of increasing their ability to withstand the debilitating aspects of stressful life
events. Prevention skillbuilding aims at equipping populations with both
the ability to effectively solve problems of daily living and to increase
tolerance for the often difficult to manage feelings associated with distressing life events. Furthermore, prevention activities are often proactive
rather than reactive (Albee, 1978; Cowen, 1978). This feature engenders
much of the enthusiasm heard among prevention practitioners. For if, in
fact, it can be demonstrated that preventive interventions directed at building coping and competency skills prior to the occurrence of natural disas-
ters, home disruptions, or other stressful life events, reduce demands for
traditional one-to-one intervention; then, primary prevention may indeed
prove to be both cost effective and a viable investment for resources for the
80s.

The purpose of this paper is to provide human service practitioners with
a model for primary prevention activity planning for the 80s. This model is
intended to provide the practitioner with the means for legitimizing the
allocation of scarce resources (i.e., dollars and personnel), for planning,
implementing, and evaluating prevention activities. The model offers a
rationale for intervention planning, a means for identifying the factors in a
group or community which may be targeted for an intervention, a formula

for assessing the current status of that group or community, and recommends strategies for evaluating the impact of the selected intervention on the targeted group or community.

This model is also useful for the evaluator whose task it may be to design measures to describe the impact of an intervention on a new group. If the guided steps to planning a prevention activity are followed, the practitioner should have set the stage for the evaluator to begin his work. The model then, can also serve as a bridging tool between the practitioner and the evaluator by serving to clarify the objectives of preventive interventions.

Assumptions of the Model

Several assumptions are inherent in the model:

1. The life span of every human being is characterized by a series of progressive, predictable developmental stages. In each of these stages, skills are expected to emerge or be developed which can eventuate in the adequate preparation of the individual for adequate functioning. In order for this psychological development to occur, certain environmental conditions need to exist.

2. If the optimal conditions for development have not existed, if skills were not mastered or developed in a chronological developmental sequence, it is possible to provide "remedial" interventions that build competency in coping with skill deficit(s).

3. That "one man's stimulus can be another man's stressor" (Hollister, 1977), i.e., that risk factors, predictable stressors and their frequency, duration, and cumulative effect, and a person's psychological ability to withstand stress must all be accounted for prior to planning and intervention.

4. The level of development reached by an individual should be viewed as dynamic rather than static. The level of adjustment that we associate with a certain level of development, is in fact, likely to fluctuate between higher and lower levels, depending upon situational differences. For example, it can be expected that an individual who has reached the stage of adulthood would not utilize magical thinking as a means of explaining the current cash flow problems in his company; yet, in the aftermath of a tornado which had just torn the roof off his home and killed his oldest child, the use of magical thinking could be expected to occur. Such regression would be viewed as normative and expected following such a severe, unpredictable event (Caplan, 1964; A. Kliman, 1979).

5. That the goal of primary prevention activities is to decrease the occurrence of mental disorder by promoting healthy coping behavior and enhancing the competency of vulnerable and normal populations (Cowen, 1976; Spivack and Shure, 1978; Goldston, 1977).

The Model Itself:

The model provides the practitioner with a framework in which to conceptualize his work and serves as a planning tool for primary prevention activities. The model is interactive; it emphasizes the relationship among risk factors, stressful life events, and vulnerability to risk and stress as it affects functionality. It is also multi-dimensional in that it takes into account more than one variable in predicting outcome. It provides a means for *identifying* risk and stress factors in a selected population, a means for *assessing* coping skills and available support systems, and a means for determining *what type(s) of preventive interventions* are most likely to promote healthy outcomes for vulnerable groups.

The model consists of four quadrants, labeled A, B, C, and D. Quadrant A[1] lists potential risks factors that may be affecting a given population. Risk factors may be grouped into four categories: physical, social/economic, environmental, and behavioral. As evidenced by the location of physical risk factors on the left side of quadrant A, these are "determined" and are not generally changeable. While social/economic, environmental and behavioral factors are more amenable to change, level and cost of effort required to create the change must be considered when actually selecting the intervention(s) to be utilized.

Quadrant B presents a list of stressful life events. The box is divided to distinguish between those stressful life events that are associated with reaching and mastering predictable developmental milestones (here the presence of stress is viewed as essential to the mastery) and those events that are situational in nature and are often accompanied by debilitating stress. As more than one stressful life event is recorded, it is important to note that the cumulative effect has been described (Albee, 1978) as rising geometrically and not in a simple additive manner.

Quadrant C presents a list of factors to consider in identifying a group's ability (or individuals in a group) to withstand the debilitating effects of stress related to risk and life events. This list is useful as an inventory of strengths and resources available to the targeted population.

Quadrant D is used to enter an assessment of predicted outcome if no

---

[1]These lists are not intended to be exhaustive, but rather suggestive and informative.

Figure 1

A Primary Prevention Model for Risk Identification
Assessment and Intervention Planning

A. RISK FACTORS		B. STRESSFUL LIFE EVENTS	
Determined	Changeable	Developmental	Situational
chronic illness	low educational status	birth of a child	changes in location, vocation,
retardation	low occupational status	attachment between mother	socialization & expectations
congenital malformations	institutional sexism	& child	natural disasters
premature birth	minority status	rapprochement crisis of	accidents
irreversible impact of toxins	substandard housing	toddlerhood	acute hospitalizations
history of poor nutrition	isolation	school entry	family disruption;
poor prenatal care	"learned helplessness"	adolescence	separation, divorce
poor health care	suggestibility	middle age	birth of a sibling
FAS syndrome	guilibility	"empty nest"	reconstituted or step families
traumatic experiences	self-defeating behaviors	retirement	adoption
		aging	child abuse
			rape
			widowhood

C. STRENGTHS & RESOURCES		D. OUTCOME ASSESSMENT OF CURRENT STATUS OF WELL-BEING	
Skills	Supports	Disease prevention intervention Indicated –	Health promotion intervention Indicated +
frustration tolerance	familial (including	-drug abuse	-responsible use of
tolerance for withstanding	extended family	-juvenile delinquency	substances
negative feelings	social	-truancy	-academic achievement
ability to problem-solve	religious	-hostile acting out	-appropriate interaction with
ability to utilize one's prior	organizational	-runaway	authority figures
experiences as resources	work-related		-positive peer group interaction
assertiveness	self-help groups		-community resource user
communication	"significant other,"		
stress management	i.e., teacher, hot		
	dog vendor, customer		
	on newpaper route		
	natural helping networks		

73

intervention were to occur. This quadrant requires the practitioner to make judgment predicting outcome based on entries for the targeted population in Quadrants A, B, and C. The model is flexible in that it does not weight one quadrant as more influential than another. Nor does it prescribe in which quadrant(s) the intervention(s) should be directed. What the model does accomplish is a clear documentation of the characteristics of the targeted population and an estimation of outcome if no intervention were to be applied.

How to Use the Model

The first task is *identification* of the risk factors, stressful life events, coping skills, and support systems available to the group selected for intervention. The major methods for identifying the categories listed above include:

1. The use of a questionnaire or survey form addressed to members of the targeted group, key informants familiar with that group, i.e., (teachers, family members). The Holmes and Rahe (1970) Social Readjustment Rating Scale is useful in determining the number of stressful events and assigning weights to them.

2. A collection of statistics on the geographic area under study.

3. Access to records, i.e., schools, courts, hospitals, birth certificates.[2]

4. A psychological interview to determine status of coping skills.

The program practitioner who systematically approaches the delivery of prevention services by identifying risk factors, stressful life events, and coping skills and resources will have provided a focus to the activity that can be evaluated and held accountable.

The second task is to examine the relationship among the risk factors, stressful life events, coping skills and support systems. This *assessment* is based on the judgment of at least two practitioners involved in this planning process. The following simple formula is suggested:

$$(CS + SS) \odot (R) \odot (S) = 0 \text{ of MH/MI}$$
(Coping Skills + Support Systems) $\odot$ Risk $\odot$ Stress
= Predicted Outcome
of Mental Health or
Mental Illness

---

[2]Ramsey (1978) at the University of North Carolina has reported his findings on predicting school failure from the birth certificate.

in which the symbol ⊙ is to be interpreted as "as they (it) relate(s) to."

This formula serves the purpose of concretizing the variables you intend to impact and the outcome(s) you anticipate if selected intervention(s) are enacted.

Planning an Intervention

Following the assessment phase, the intervention planning cycle begins. Preventive interventions are activities that are aimed at affecting a positive outcome in a population that has been determined as vulnerable to the development of mental disorder in the assessment process. The vulnerability may be temporary, i.e., due to a situational stress, and the intervention may be stress specific and short in duration. The vulnerability may also be long-standing and require long-term planning and follow through.

Preventive interventions can be of several types: They may include environmental manipulation (Reinherz, 1980), parent education, community education, promotion and formation of support groups, and providing access to community programs (i.e., YMCA, Meals on Wheels). They may involve the validation of the legitimacy of reactions to stressful situations, the sharing of solutions, the provision of supportive services.

In planning an intervention, it is essential that the factors to be impacted be specified and documented. Figure 2 depicts various options in intervention planning.

Preventive Interventions may be aimed at:

1. Reducing risk factor(s) and thus increasing mental health status.

2. Managing and diluting stress associated with mastery of predictable developmental events and situational events and thus increasing or maintaining mental health status.

3. Increasing coping and competency skills and increasing or maintaining mental health status.

4. Increasing support systems and increasing or maintaining mental health status.

A Worksheet for Planning Primary Prevention Activities

The following worksheet was designed[3] to provide practitioners and evaluators with specific guidelines for utilizing the model and moving from

[3]The worksheet was prepared and used by Forquer, S.L., Kamis, E., Newman, F.L.; Eastern Pennsylvania Psychiatric Institute as part of NIMH Region IV Contract #140-0079-17, Technical Assistance in Primary Prevention for Community Mental Health Centers in the State of Tennessee. An example of this application is available from the author.

FIGURE 2

Variations in Intervention Planning and Outcome Measurements

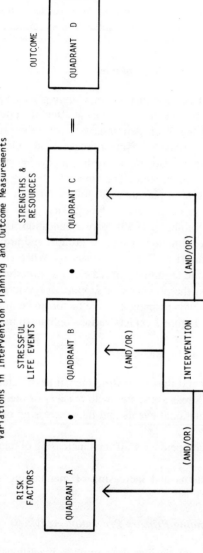

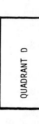

Forquer, 1980

I. Interventions can be directed at either A, B, or C or a combination of A, B, C.

II. Following the intervention(s), changes are anticipated in: OUTCOME

as a result of changes in Cells A, B and/or C.

76

identification to assessment to intervention planning to evaluation of the prevention activity and its impact.

1. *Name* the target population and others who would indirectly benefit from potential intervention.

2. *Identify* both the direct and indirect populations in terms of risk factors, demographic characteristics, neighborhood characteristics.

3. *Identify* risk factors, major stress(es), strengths (coping skills), and assets (support) affecting the target population. List in Quadrants A, B, and C of the model.

4. *Assess* the vulnerability of the target group, using the formula (CS + SS) $\odot$ (R) $\odot$ (S) = 0. Enter prediction without intervention in Quadrant D of the model.

5. *Define* what problems or major disabling factors within the target population you wish to reduce or eliminate. State what existing strengths you plan to utilize and what competencies you plan to increase. Enter an outcome cell *with* intervention in the model. Indicate what factors you plan to effect.

6. *Establish* one or more short and long term working objectives.

7. *Decide* who needs to be involved in working toward objectives, i.e., board of directors, administration, other community groups.

8. *Design* the steps to be taken to secure the interest and cooperation of those in Item #6.

9. Now *outline* an achievable program. Include activities and actors, tasks, task goals, time frames, and resources.

10. *Design* record keeping and activity documentation.

11. *Specify* and evaluation strategy in terms of procedures, time frame, process, and outcome measures.

12. *Build* in feedback procedures, including those involved in #6.

13. *Determine* format for final report including evaluation, recommended modification, and dissemination strategy.

14. Is funding needed? What level? What sources can be approached?

REFERENCES

Albee, G. A systems approach to primary prevention. Presented at St. Francis Community Mental Health Center, Pittsburgh, Pennsylvania, February 1, 1978.

Caplan, G. *Principles of Preventive Psychiatry.* New York: Basic Books, Inc., 1964.

Cowen, E.L. Some problems in community program evaluation research. *Journal of Consulting and Clinical Psychology.* 1978, Vol. 46 (4), 792–805.

Hollister, W.G. Basic strategies in designing primary prevention programs. In Klein, D.C.

and Goldston, S. (Eds.). *Primary Prevention: An Idea Whose Time Has Come*, National Institute of Mental Health, Maryland, 1977, pp. 41–48.

Holmes, T. and Rahe. Social readjustment rating scale. In *Human Behavior: Stress*. Chicago: Time-Life Books, 1970.

Kliman, A.S. *Crisis—Psychological first aid for recovery* and *growth*. New York: Holt, Rinehart and Winston, 1978.

Mahler, M.S.: Pine, F; and Bergman, A. *The Psychological birth of the human infant*. New York: Basic Books, Inc., 1975.

President's Commission on Mental Health. *Report* to the *President*, Vol. 1. Washington, D.C.: U.S. Government Printing Office, 1978.

Ramey, C.T., Stedman, D.S., Borders-Patterson, A., & Mengel, W. Predicting school failure from information available at birth. *American Journal of Mental Deficiency*, 1978, *82*, 525–534.

Reinherz, H. Primary prevention of emotional disorders of children: Mirage or reality. *Journal of Prevention*, Vol. 1 (1), 1980.

Shure, M.B. and Spivack, G. *Problem-Solving techniques in childrearing*. Jossey-Bass Publishers, San Francisco: 1978.

COMMUNITY EDUCATION

REACHING TARGET POPULATIONS WITH PREVENTIVE MENTAL HEALTH EDUCATION PROGRAMS

Iris Nahemow, PhD

ABSTRACT. This brief article contains suggested strategies for recruiting participants in Preventive Mental Health Education Programs.

The old story about the donkey which ends . . . ". . . but first you have to get his attention!" depicts the problem of mental health educators implementing their well conceptualized, beautifully developed, and obviously important programs in the community. Graduate programs in child development don't include marketing courses and so we often struggle to reach our target population with information about our prevention programs. Some of the ideas that worked for one agency follow. Perhaps they may work for others.

Planning

1. Before beginning to market your program, know whom you wish to reach.
2. Use an advisory group comprised of members of your target population. They can help you identify: (a) what they read—place articles and ads here; (b) where your group goes—this is the place for posters; (c) what

Iris Nahemow, PhD, is Director of Consultation and Education at Allegheny East MH/MR Center, Inc., Suite 400, Monroeville Medical Arts Building, 2550 Mosside Boulevard, Monroeville, PA 15146.

language appeals to them—use it in your brochures and fliers; (d) to whom they talk—these folks can be important referral sources.

3. Is an appropriate mailing list available? Use it for a bulk mailing!

Activities

1. Begin with articles in local newspapers. A call to the feature editor will often result in a large FREE article with accompanying photos. Feature editors need fresh ideas for each edition of the paper, and are well worth cultivating.

2. Use public service announcements in newspapers, and local radio and TV stations to publicize your program.

3. Place small paid (or free, if possible) ads in the classified section of your newspaper. Repeat for three to four weeks.

4. Develop brochures and fliers to place in grocery stores, childrens shops, toy stores, and laundromats. Use posters for community bulletin boards. (Check with your advisory committee. They will know if your language and format are appealing.)

5. Create a mailing list by asking attendees at public groups and talks if they'd like to be included.

6. Use a list from birth announcements, pre-schools, baby photographers, or similar sources to mail fliers directly to homes. (Your program participants will add names of their friends, too.)

7. Visit or mail notices to pre-schools, clergy, and pediatricians asking that they publicize your programs.

Each of these activities must be repeated many times and each reinforces the others. People need to see your name repeatedly for best results.

Evaluation

1. At registration, ask each person how they heard about the program. Keep records of this to help during your next planning period.

2. Ask your participants for additional ways of publicizing your programs. You may be pleasantly surprised by the effectiveness of their suggestions.

Good programs deserve good marketing. This is the way the community learns that a needed service is available. Remember that it takes time and much trial and error for an organization to find the best combination of activities for reaching its targeted group. Good luck!

TRAINING PROGRAMS

EDUCATING PRACTITIONERS
IN PRIMARY PREVENTION

Karen VanderVen, PhD

ABSTRACT. This paper describes reasons for lags in preparation of primary prevention manpower, some primary prevention activities along with knowledge, skills, and attributes necessary to implement them, and implications for educational programs and activities.

"Interfering with effective preventive programs is the *serious shortage of well-qualified people prepared to work and plan in this area* (Albee, 1980, p. 8). To address this problem, it is necessary to consider reasons for lags in education of primary prevention manpower, core primary prevention activities, and the knowledge, skills, and attributes necessary to conduct them, and the overall implications for educational programs and activities in primary prevention.

Failure to Educate Practitioners in Primary Prevention Skills

It seems quite well established in the history of mental health service and treatment that interventions have focused on intrapsychic processes of the individual rather than the larger systems containing and affecting him. "Mental health agencies, while acknowledging the *logical* importance of primary prevention, continue to devote their major resources to diagnosis,

---

Karen VanderVen, PhD, is Associate Professor, Child Development and Child Care, School of Health Related Professions, University of Pittsburgh, Pittsburgh, PA 15261.

treatment, and rehabilitation, and neglect the serious implementation of preventative interventions'' (Broskowski and Baker, 1974, p. 708). "People are attracted to psychiatry, psychology, social work, nursing and the other mental health professions in significant part because of the high visibility of a 'treatment philosophy', a *commitment to a one to one intervention*'' (Albee, 1980, p. 6).

Thus, it is not surprising that the educational preparation of psychiatrists (Klerman and Levinson, 1969; Harrison and Delano, 1976), social workers (Patti and Austin, 1977), and child care practitioners (VanderVen, 1979, 1980, 1981) focuses primarily on the development of clinical, direct line skills, rather than including preparation for the different types of skills required to conduct primary prevention activities. Therefore, a block to primary prevention "has been the lack of manpower specifically trained in theory and practice for carrying out primary prevention . . ." (Broskowski and Baker, 1974, p. 708). This general situation may be accounted for in part by the ideology that mental problems and developmental lags are caused from within the individual and require individual treatment for amelioration (Albee, 1980). As a result, many practitioners may have neither the orientation nor the skills to assume roles in primary prevention activities which focus on changing systems rather than individuals and which generally are timed earlier than individual treatment interventions. When practitioners have moved into work in the wider caregiving system, required to serve as administrators, consultants, program planners, and similar functions, they have not been prepared to perform them. As a result, their potential to achieve real impact has been diminished.

Child Ecology as a Rationale for Education in Primary Prevention

The formulations of Bronfenbrenner (1977, 1979) concerning the impact on children of the hierarchical levels in a total ecological system provides a strong rationale for the relevance of primary prevention in promoting children's positive development and mental health, and ultimately, for the educational preparation of practitioners with primary prevention skills. The microsystem, the first ecological level, is the immediate environment containing a child; events in the microsystem include relationships among persons in the setting, the activities conducted in the setting, and its physical features. The next two levels, the mesosystem and exosystems, include the relationships among the major settings containing the person, and among settings that do not actually contain him, but affect and even determine what takes place in them. The top ecological level consists of "the overarching institutional patterns of the culture or subculture such as the economic, social, legal, and political systems. . ." (Bronfenbrenner, 1977, p. 515).

That ecological, or social environmental factors are strong influences on the lives of children is also supported by Cowen:

> People's (especially children's) development and adaptation are significantly shaped by a limited number of high-impact social environments: Communities, churches, schools, and families. In the past, we have tended to take properties of these systems for granted and, except for so intimate a system as the family, to overlook their shaping impact (Cowen, p. 12).

Traditional treatment and interventive approaches have focused primarily on the activities of the microsystem, most specifically on the interpersonal relationships within it. Thus, the additional options of intervening in, or affecting the physical environment and the activities within it, thus providing a stronger impact, have not been taken. The other three levels, the mesosystem, exosystem, and macrosystem, are minimally affected by these approaches.

Primary prevention activities, on the other hand, have a tremendous potential to make an impact on the multilevel systems influencing the quality of children's lives and development because they are targeted on these systems. However, many of the skills required for primary prevention are quite different from those involved in direct care in the microsystem. They are skills in indirect practice which are not delivered to clients in direct contact, but rather are oriented towards influencing the wider systems that contain and strongly affect them. Educational preparation of mental health practitioners must include indirect skills if at least some workers are to be able to function effectively in a primary prevention mode.

Core Activities of Primary Prevention and Related Professional Skills

To propose educational activities for persons to serve in the indirect systems approach of primary prevention requires the explication of some of the core activities subsumed under the concept of primary prevention for children and deriving from these the educational suggestions.

Early Childhood Intervention

In line with the premise that the earlier the preventive effort, the more likely it will be able to serve a primary prevention function. Therefore, early childhood programs play a particularly significant role. Early intervention into child rearing practices (Bloom, 1979), provision of environmental supports for families and children, and specific facilitation of social, emotional, and cognitive development, can prevent the later entrenchment of educational and adjustment problems. Prenatal programs, parent-child programs, parent education programs, preschool programs such as Head Start, and similar activities can be viewed as mental health programs (Glasscote and Fishman, 1974) with a primary prevention function. In early childhood intervention, direct as well as indirect skills are necessary. Knowledge of basic child development is essential in education for primary prevention (Goldston, 1977). In addition, a wide spectrum of skills necessary to develop and actually conduct programs is needed and would include interpersonal and community relationships, environmental design, instruction of children and adults, crisis intervention, program planning, coordination, evaluation, and organizational design.

Mental Health Promotion

A major aspect of primary prevention has been conceptualized as health promotion (Bloom, 1979; Eisenberg, 1979). This is congruent with current trends in work with children. For young children, there is an interesting orientation towards actively teaching them cognitive problem solving skills so that they can better cope with and actually positively influence their own environments. This is in some contrast with the more traditional perspectives that favor more passive approaches and assume that such young children can only be the recipients of environmental transactions. The work of Spivack and Shure (1977) exemplifies the newer mode which is more in line with the primary prevention philosophy.

With older children who have been identified as having specific behavioral and emotional problems, the contemporary perspective favors development of skills and competence through an educative approach as contrasted to only orienting treatment towards amelioration of specific pathological syndromes (Hobbs, 1974; Whittaker, 1979). Both of these approaches to children of different age groups can be viewed as mental health promotion. Related skills for the practitioner would include knowledge of problem solving strategies, a wide variety of childhood activities, and teaching.

Facilitating Environments

Despite the tremendous amount of knowledge of the relationship between physical environments and human behavior (Moos, 1975); and the recognition of the significance of the physical environment as a factor in primary prevention (Forgays, Ed., 1978), much of this does not seem to have been applied in actual practice. Even though, in many children's settings, there may be claims about a "therapeutic milieu" or a "learning environment," scrutiny suggests that they are in fact unstimulating and actually discouraging of the kind of behavior they are supposedly facilitating. Thus, skill in the structuring of time and space, and knowledge of the dimensions of the therapeutic milieu or developmental setting, are crucial for the primary prevention practitioner.

Psychological Aspects of Physical Conditions

While the public health base of primary prevention has focused on the prevention of specific diseases, a growing aspect of primary prevention in mental health is on the prevention of emotional problems which can result from physical conditions if not given early or concomitant attention. Thus, for children, there are now "child life" programs providing emotional support for hospitalized children, discussion groups for parents of children suffering various physical impairments, and treatment activities to help the children deal with their feelings generated by their conditions. The growing field of pediatric psychology (Roberts, Queuillon, Wright, 1979) provides the knowledge base for these activities; practitioners must know the characteristics of various children's diseases and physical impairments, the nature of their possible emotional sequelae, and, particularly, of programmatic approaches that can be brought to bear to address them. The idea of making emotionally-focused interventions is quite new to many traditional health settings; thus the practitioners must know the dynamics of such settings and strategies for changing them.

Organizational Dynamics

The structure and dynamics of the organizations that deliver various human services are particularly significant in primary prevention (Bolman,

1979). Although planning and coordination are key aspects of work within an organizational context, many practitioners do not have skills in these and thus "planning remains piecemeal and coordination is token. Prevention has no real clout" (Bolman, 1979, p. 10). The implications for the education of primary prevention practitioners is obvious: they must have skills appropriate for working effectively in the organizational systems found at all levels of the ecological hierarchy. These would include, in addition to general planning and coordination, goal and objective setting, delegation, communication, team building, collaboration, negotiation, evaluation, budgeting, and consultation. Consultation is a particular skill utilized in primary prevention efforts and one in which the practitioner must be trained, in line with Lachenmeyer: "the actual work of the consultant may differ in some respects from the ways in which he or she has been trained" (in Gibbs, Lachenmeyer, Sigal, eds., 1980, p. 271).

Specific program design skills are also part of the organizational skills requirement of the primary preventionist. The degree to which the practitioner can establish sound objectives, preferably based on a needs assessment and addressing relevant variables in the various levels of the ecological hierarchy of influences on children; the degree to which they can be translated into effective activities, and to the explication of appropriate staff and resources necessary to conduct them, are all related to the ultimate impact of the program.

Community Focus

Congruent with the ecological rationale for primary prevention is its community, as contrasted to individual focus. Rather than targeting efforts towards specific individuals, primary prevention requires broader based work with the structure and dynamics of the community, so that needs of wider populations can be identified and encompassing interventions can be designed. For this to take place, practitioners must have knowledge of the economic, employment, housing, health, educational, religious, recreational, and many other major institutions of the community; and their relationship to mental health. Most specifically, they need to know how to organize to achieve changes in those institutions that do not serve people's mental health needs. For example, an inner city adolescent can discuss his despair at being unable to find a job or appropriate job training with an empathic counselor. But the only true way out of his dilemma will be the actual alteration of the employment and educational systems of his community. This is no mean task but is definitely crucial to be effective in a true primary prevention mode.

Facilitating Development of Primary Prevention Manpower Through Education

As has been described, a wide variety of non-traditional roles are required for mental health practitioners to assume primary prevention functions. Specific content and knowledge required to do this has been stated. There are some additional considerations. Studies of professional development of clinicians in various disciplines suggest that the job roles in both direct and indirect work are related to the particular stage of adult development that they are in. Those roles which require more complex skills or ability to conceptualize are, of course, most likely to be effectively filled by more seasoned, mature practitioners. This suggests that some of the mandates of primary prevention require that practitioners be able to function in a way congruent with greater experience and maturity. For example, to be able to recognize the relationship between organizational factors and the quality of direct service requires the cognitive maturity to be able to identify with service givers as well as clients, and to recognize the complexities of interactions among various aspects of relevant systems. Categorical thinking has been identified as serving as a barrier to primary prevention (Bolman, 1979) and also, as "non-synergistic" thinking, as being characteristic of human service practitioners in their initial stages of career development (King and VanderVen, 1978). If experience and evolving maturity are necessary in order to view things from a variety of perspectives, rather than categorically, then the educational system needs to respond. First of all, it can provide some exposure to indirect modes of practice to students in initial professional preparation so that they can have a basis for seeing these functions as relevant and worthy to consider. Secondly, through both content and attitude, it should facilitate the development of mature cognitive skills. Systems approaches and a variety of perspectives and approaches should be taught. There should be ample opportunity for practice in problem solving in a variety of situations and settings. Specific sequences in primary prevention—in depth—might be offered at a later time in professional preparation after the practitioner has acquired some direct line experience in microsystem settings and has advanced in his/her own development as an adult.

REFERENCES

Adams, M. The compassion trap. In V. Gornick and M. Moran (Eds.) *Woman in sexist society*. New York: Basic Books, 1971.
Albee, G. W. A brief historical perspective on the primary prevention of childhood mental disorders. Unpublished paper, University of Vermont, undated.

Albee, G. W. Proceedings of the annual Gisela Konopka Lectureship. Center for Youth Development and Research, University of Minnesota, May 21, 1980.

Albee, G. W., & Joffe, J. M. *Primary prevention of psychopathology, Vol. 1.* Hanover, New Hampshire: The University Press of New England, 1977.

Bloom, B. L. Prevention of mental disorders: Recent advances in theory and practice. *Community Mental Health Journal,* 1979, *15,* 179-191.

Bolman, W. Obstacles to prevention. In J. Noshpitz (Ed.), *The basic handbook of child psychiatry,* Vol. IV., *Prevention and current issues.* New York: Basic Books, 1979.

Bronfenbrenner, U. *The ecology of human development: Experiments by nature and design.* Cambridge: Harvard University Press, 1979.

Bronfenbrenner, U. Toward an experimental ecology of human development. *American Psychologist,* 1977, *32,* 513-530.

Broskowski, A., & Schulberg, H. C. A model training program for clinical research and development. *Professional Psychology, 5,* 133-139.

Broskowski, A., & Baker, F. Professional, organizational, and social barriers to primary prevention. *American Journal of Orthopsychiatry,* 1974, *44,* 707-719.

Coan, R. W. *Psychologists: Personal and theoretical pathways.* New York: Irvington Publishers, Inc., 1979.

Cowen, E. L. Demystifying primary prevention. In D. G. Forgays (Ed.), *Primary prevention of psychopathology, Vol. 2.* Hanover, New Hampshire: The University Press of New England, 1978.

Davids, A. Therapeutic approaches to children in residential treatment. *American Psychologist,* 1975, *32,* 809-814.

Eisenberg, L. Introduction—Preventive methods in psychiatry: Definitions, principles and social politics. In J. Noshpitz (Ed.), *The basic handbook of child psychiatry, Vol. IV, Prevention and current issues.* New York: Basic Books, 1969.

Forgays, D. G. (Ed.) *Primary prevention of psychopathology. Vol. 2.* Hanover, New Hampshire: The University Press of New England, 1978.

Gibbs, M. S., Lachenmeyer, J. R., & Sigal, J. (Eds.) *Community psychology.* New York: Gardner Press, Inc., 1980.

Glasscote, R., & Fishman, M. E. *Mental health programs for preschool children.* American Psychiatric Association, 1974.

Goldston, S. Defining primary prevention. In G. W. Albee and J. M. Joffe (Eds.), *Primary prevention of psychopathology. Vol. 1.* Hanover, New Hampshire: The University Press of New England, 1977.

Harrison, S. I., & Delano, J. G. The status of prevention in the education of child psychiatrists. *Child Psychiatry and Human Development,* 1976, *7,* 3-21.

Hinkle, A., & Burns, M. The clinician-executive: A review. *Administration in Mental Health,* 1978, *6,* 3-21.

Hobbs, N. Helping disturbed children. In M. Wolins (Ed.), *Successful group care.* Chicago: Aldine, 1974.

King, M., & VanderVen, K. Personal development and values of child care practitioners. *Creative Child and Adult Quarterly,* 1978, *5,* 2.

Klerman, G., & Levinson, D. Becoming the director: Promotion as a phase in personal-professional development. *Psychiatry,* 1969, *32,* 411-427.

Lachenmeyer, J. Mental health consultation and programmatic change. In M. Gibbs, J. R. Lachenmeyer, and J. Sigal (Eds.) *Community psychology.* New York: Gardner Press, Inc., 1980.

Moos, R. *The human context: Environmental determinants of behavior.* New York: John Wiley, 1976.

Noshpitz, J., Ed. *The basic handbook of child psychiatry, Vol. IV., Prevention and current issues.* New York: Basic Books, 1969.

Patti, R., & Austin, M. Socializing the direct service practitioner in the ways of supervisory management. *Administration in Social Work,* 1977, *1,* 267–280.

Roberts, M., Queuillon, R., & Wright, L. Pediatric psychology: A developmental report and survey of the literature. *Child and Youth Services,* 1979, *2,* 1–9.

Spivack, G., & Shure, M. Preventively oriented cognitive education of preschoolers. In D. Klein and S. Goldston (Eds.), *Primary prevention: An idea whose time has come.* Washington, D.C.: U.S. Government Printing Office. DHEW Pub. No. (ADM) 77-447, 1977.

VanderVen, K. Facilitating personal and professional development of child care practitioners for new roles in group care. In *New directions in group care.* London: Tavistock Press. To be published 1981.

VanderVen, K. A paradigm describing stages of personal and professional development of child care practitioners with characteristics associated with each stage. *Proceedings of the 9th International Congress of the International Association of Workers with Maladjusted Children.* Montreal, Canada, 1980.

VanderVen, K. Developmental characteristics of child care workers and design of training programs. *Child Care Quarterly,* 1979, *8,* 100–112.

Whittaker, J. *Caring for troubled children.* San Francisco: Jossey Bass, 1979.

PREVENTION: PROMISE OR PREMISE?
A TRAINING PROGRAM
IN THE PRIMARY PREVENTION
OF CHILDHOOD MENTAL DISORDERS

Ruth P. Kane, MD
Evelyn Wiszinckas, PhD
Sandra L. Forquer, PhD

ABSTRACT. This is a report on an NIMH-funded three year training and demonstration program in the primary prevention of childhood mental disorders for caregivers. Strategies for recruitment of participants, implementation, and evaluation are described. Two major issues are addressed: (a) success in meeting and maintaining initial recruitment objectives and (b) the nature of program impact on participants. The report concludes that the program has been successful in both meeting and maintaining recruitment objectives and in demonstrating positive impact upon program participants. Positive impact has been measured by increase in knowledge, job application, and program implementation. Implications for future program replications are discussed.

Dr. Ruth P. Kane is Director, Children and Adolescent Mental Health Services and Chief of Consultation Education Services, St. Francis General Hospital, Mental Health/Mental Retardation Center, 45 and Penn Avenue, Pittsburgh, PA 15201, and Clinical Associate Professor of Child Psychiatry, University of Pittsburgh. Evelyn Wiszinckas is Project Director of Primary Prevention Training Program for Caregivers, St. Francis General Hospital. Sandra Forquer is former Project Director of Primary Prevention Training Program for Caregivers, St. Francis General Hospital, Pittsburgh, PA.

Introduction

Prevention of mental disorder has been an ideal of the mental health movement since its inception in the early 1900's. In order to disseminate concepts of primary prevention to community caregivers, particularly as applied to childhood mental disorders, training them in its principle and practice seemed to be a reasonable way to proceed. Primary prevention can be looked upon as involving those efforts aimed at reducing the incidence of mental disorders according to Caplan (1961) or in terms of health promotion according to Bloom (1979). Prior to the training program, St. Francis General Hospital Mental Health Mental Retardation Center had been engaged in a number of outreach projects through a Part F NIMH Grant # 03-H-001, 715-08 on Primary Prevention and Early Intervention of Childhood Mental Disorders in Children from 0-8 years. As part of these endeavors as well as other community outreach programs by the Consultation Education Services of St. Francis General Hospital Community Mental Health Center, contacts had been established with a variety of Human Services workers including Mental Health workers, Health Care Systems, Educational Systems, and Welfare Systems prior to the training program. Because mental health services per se and particularly in the area of children and adolescent services are very meager in rural areas, training was offered to trainees in several areas—urban, suburban, and rural.

Description of the Training Program
in Primary Prevention of Mental Disorders

In July, 1977, St. Francis General Hospital Community Mental Health Center in Pittsburgh, Pennsylvania, was awarded a three year grant from the National Institute of Mental Health (#5715 19H 15012-03) to provide a training program in the primary prevention of childhood mental disorders for community caregivers. Community caregivers were recruited from three counties—Allegheny, with largely urban and some suburban areas; Westmoreland, which is rural, some poverty in some middle class areas; and Butler, which is rural and generally isolated. The program was designed to provide seminars and workshops presented by national as well as local experts in primary prevention to a variety of levels of trainees from paraprofessionals to professionals who dealt with children and their families in the tri-county area. The overall goal of the program was to provide caregivers with knowledge and skills and to enhance their positive attitudes towards goals of primary prevention in the areas of childhood and adolescent mental health and retardation services.

Program Design

The program had two basic objectives. The first was to gain and maintain a commitment of a group of trainees from multidisciplinary backgrounds to a three year program. The second objective was to deliver a program which would have impact on participants as measured by increased knowledge, job application, and program implementation. Dissemination of the training program package was earmarked as a third objective in the final year.

1. *Commitment.* The first program objective was to recruit and maintain continuous participation of the trainees in the program.

2. *Impact.* The second objective was to provide curriculum content and consultation that would increase trainees knowledge of primary prevention, provide skills that could be applied to their daily work, and supply trainees with combinations of skills and knowledge necessary to design and implement preventive projects. (a) *Knowledge.* enabled participants to distinguish programs which have primary preventive focus from those which offer secondary and tertiary prevention; promoting awareness of current delivery system models; and providing theoretical framework in child development and primary prevention and different life stages. Ideas were to delineate predictable as well as unpredictable crises. (b) *Application.* to provide skills to increase participants ability. (c) *Implementation.* to provide knowledge and skills that would enable them to design and implement projects.

3. The third objective was to disseminate training packages and primary prevention beyond tri-county area in evaluation procedures implemented to see where indeed the objectives and goals had been met in the training program.

Meeting the Program Objectives

Recruitment and Commitment

The St. Francis General Hospital Community Mental Health Mental Retardation Center had an extensive history of community involvement both with direct and indirect service. Ongoing relationships with agencies serving children had been established since the maintenance of children's outpatient and inpatient services in 1966 and 1968 respectively. Consultation Education efforts in primary prevention with caregivers of children and families from 0–8 years at risk for mental disorders were provided by the Part F NIMH Grant #03-H-001, 715-08. Initial strategies were developed in order to recruit caregivers from multidisciplinary backgrounds for this training program. A project director was selected who had knowledge of the Children's Mental Health Services at St. Francis General Hospital and ongoing relationships with agencies and caregivers in the tricounty area.

Agencies selected in addition to those known to the Project Director were selected by the following strategies. A high level representative from each agency to be recruited was invited to participate on the Advisory Board of the Grant. These representatives gave input regarding missing pieces of the system to be trained. Visits were then made to the agencies to be recruited.

Trainee selections were made by the criteria of the agency sending the trainees itself and by the stipulation that some of the trainees would be in a position to enable them to train others in their own agencies. Recruitment was also made on the basis of trainees having already a considerable commitment to the agency and desire to stay on at the agency. The number of trainees per agency depended on the size of the agency and the county they represented. The third strategy used was developing and administering a Needs Assessment. This provided agency directors and potential trainees with a vehicle through which to add input to the curriculum content of the program. The Needs Assessment had two purposes, first to serve and foster continuous participation of trainees, and secondly, to insure that the programs offered would meet not only program requirements and needs of trainees, but also needs of directors and administrators of participating agencies.

In order to insure training commitment, ongoing responsiveness to trainee needs was employed. Trainee feedback regarding program content, format and other program issues were actively sought throughout the three year program. This was done both formally and informally. As much as possible, adjustments were made to meet perceived needs and suggestions.

Evaluation

Evaluation of recruitment and commitment were made by several measures. These were attendance records and group composition data which was regularly compiled and analyzed. Trainees responsiveness to the program was assessed through a consumer satisfaction and evaluation form distributed at the end of each session and through annual personal interviews with each trainee.

Results of recruitment and commitment was originally from those who took a knowledge and skills pretest utilizing case examples called Pretest

181. By year three, 112 were still in the program. Only 156 of the 181 people actually attended at least one subsequent training session. These were called the original trainees. Other possible participating trainees who took part in the personal interviews refer to years one, two and three. More of the trainees came from Allegheny County. County representation remained stable for the duration of the program. A slight decrease was observed in urban representation and a slight increase in suburban and rural. Systems involved were health care, social service, education, health education, and clergy. At the end of the program there was a slight decrease in health care, maintenance of the same percentage in social service, an increase in education, a slight increase in health education, and a decrease in clergy. Professional level representation went from upper level administrative, middle level administrative, to direct service, academic, and student. The upper level administrators were about the same at the end of their training program (8 to 10%), middle level administrators increasing, direct service had the largest number slight decrease, academic about the same at the end of the program, and students about the same. Trainees were from direct service and middle administrative levels. Educational levels showed the people were from multi-education background, the majority having a masters or bachelors degree, a few high school graduates, RNs, and the smallest number of PhD and physicians. The composition remained for the most part stable through the three years of the program in spite of variability in individual representation.

The analysis of attrition from 156 in the first year to 112 in the third year was as follows. The 112 remaining in year three were not all the same people who were the original trainees, as some people left the program they were replaced by others. The original trainees who left the program at the end of year two were identified and contacted and asked to state reasons for leaving, and the same from year three. Reasons for leaving were: (1) demands of work; (2) course ending; (3) relocation; (4) job loss; and (5) new employer. Satisfaction and ability to apply material were cited as secondary reasons by 11 out of 90 trainees who left, which suggests that the program was perceived as useful even by those who did leave. The attrition rate of the 90 who left showed that they represented 58% of the original trainees.

Attendance analysis showed that the number of people attending the sessions varied. Hazardous weather conditions in winter months were associated with low attendance at sessions one and eleven. Analysis of the attendance data suggests (a) program strategy of having prominent professionals as speakers was successful in attracting participants to these sessions; (b) specific contact areas directly related to interventive application was most effective in attracting participants; and (c) when a prominent speaker returned for a second presentation, attendance was lowered as compared with their first attendance unless the topic was very different. It was seen that in the initial recruitment efforts a result in training group of 27% regular attenders during the course of the three year program occurred.

Assessing the impact of program objectives first involved planning of curriculum content following collection of data received from needs assessment. A meeting was held with the Advisory Board and a format developed that would address educational needs identified by the assessment in programmed ideas held by the project staff. The curriculum content was divided into five specific phases to provide trainees with the framework and time table for learning processes that they were undertaking. The strategy was to utilize nationally known persons who had expertise in primary prevention in the large group, and another strategy was the use of small group process in the afternoon to digest the material and promote interchange and link-up of the varying systems who were participating in the conference. County meetings were also held once a month in addition to training sessions to encourage networking and linkage. Afternoon workshops followed a more formal morning presentation after training sessions to allow for small group exploration of the particular facet of the session. Personal interviews conducted at the end of each year served as evaluations and vehicles for providing trainees personal contact with the Director and helped act as a motivator for continuing participation in the primary prevention programs. Expertise from the Hospital Public Relations Office in designing program brochures also helped. Some trainees were offered credits for continuing education college—credits of Bachelors, Masters, and Post Masters level were offered. Certificates for the number of hours of training completed were given by the Hospital.

Measures of Impact

Several measures of impact were designed—these were: formal testing to test knowledge and skills developed with the assistance of Norman Mulgrave, PhD, of the Division of Educational Studies of the University of Pittsburgh. A test was designed to assess the impact of content in the first two program years. The same test was readministered in the third program year to assess the impact of material. A practicum option was offered to trainees in the third program year where they were offered staff assistance in developing a prevention program of their own. Personal interviews were

SPECIFIC PHASES OF PROGRAMS IN PRIMARY PREVENTION

PHASE I January-June 1978	PHASE II September-December 1978	PHASE III January-May 1979	PHASE IV September-December 1979	PHASE V January-May 1980
OBJECTIVES ●Overview of Primary Prevention ●Systems View of Primary Prevention ●A Primary Prevention Viewpoint of Child Development	OBJECTIVES ●Primary Prevention & Specific Maladaptive Syndromes of Childhood ●Primary Prevention & Specific Abnormal Crises of Childhood	OBJECTIVES ●Intervention Strategies	OBJECTIVES ●Presentation of a Conceptual Framework for Systems Entry ●Skill Acquisition in Program Development & Program Implementing	OBJECTIVES ●Consolidation of Theoretical & Practical Issues in Primary Prevention Program Development
PROGRAMS 1. "A Theoretical Overview of Primary Prevention" Gilbert Kliman, M.D.	PROGRAMS 1. "The Child in the Alcoholic Family" Abraham J. Twerski, M.D.	PROGRAMS 1. "Promoting the Mental Health of Children in the Hospital: An Opportunity for Primary Prevention" Stephen E. Goldston, Ed.D.	PROGRAMS 1. "Systems Overview & Guides to Implementation" Marshall Swift, Ph.D.	PROGRAMS 1. "A Closer Look at Family Crises: Divorce, Separation" Erna Furman
2. "A Systems Approach to Primary Prevention" George Albee, Ph.D.	2. "Children's Encounters with Death & Bereavement" Erna Furman	2. "The Nature of Problem-Solving and its Application for Primary Prevention with the Preschool Child" George Spivack, Ph.D. Myrna B. Shure, Ph.D.	2. "Program Design: Needs Assessment, Developing Goals, Program Evaluation" Norman Mulgrave, Ph.D. Thomas Whalen Shirley Dumpman Kathryn Healey, Ph.D.	2. "Primary Prevention Skills Development Day" Sandra Forquer, Ph.D. Evelyn Wiszinckas, Ph.D.
3. "A Family Approach to Primary Prevention" Ann Kliman, M.A.	3. "Primary Prevention & Child Abuse - The Victim & the Victimizer" John B. Reinhart, M.D.	3. "An Overview of the the Primary Mental Health Project" Emory Cowen, Ph.D. "Interpersonal Cognitive Problem - Solving with School-Aged Children" Ellis Gesten, Ph.D.	3. "A Grant Writing Workshop" Elizabeth Kameen Alice Kunia	3. "Child Abuse & Parental Competence" William Scheurer, Ph.D.
4. "Signs of Vulnerability in Transitional Phases (Turning, Standing Up, Walking): Helping Mothers & Children to Overcome Them" Judith Kestenberg, M.D.	4. "Primary Prevention & the Handicapped Child" Seymour Sarason, Ph.D.	4. "Immigration Neurosis & Immigration Panic: How to Help Adolescents Get Through It" Fritz Redl, Ph.D.	4. "A Demonstration in Primary Prevention Program Design" Ann Kliman, M.A.	4. "A Paradigm for the Future" G. Albee, Ph.D.
5. A Program of Active Intervention for Children Having Difficulty Adapting to Day Care" Rex Speers, M.D.		5. "Psycho-social Dimensions of Adolescent Pregnancy" Doris Welcher, Ph.D.		
6. "A Problem-Solving Approach to Primary Prevention & the School-Aged Child" Irving Berlin, M.D.				

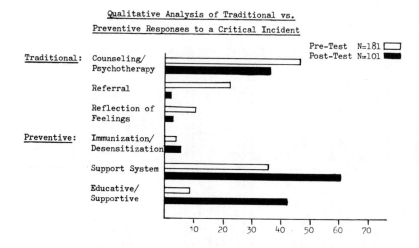

Qualitative Analysis of Traditional vs.
Preventive Responses to a Critical Incident

designed to get information about direct application of materials to the trainees in their ongoing job situations and how much trainees could implement preventive programs within their own systems. Consumer satisfaction was obtained by a form in which they rated quality of morning and afternoon sessions. The results of the pretest given at the beginning of the program and again at the end of the year of training reflects considerable increase in primary prevention knowledge and skills for trainees taking the test. The pretest score was 27, whereas the Means post-test was 43. Increase in Means group score of 15 score points. The significance of this increase in Means scores is apparent when data from the 60 trainees who took both pre and post tests were analyzed. Means test scores for the trainees who stayed in the program the first two years increased from 27 to 45. Analysis by T-Test of the difference between Means reveals 18 point increase in scores which is highly significant $P = 001$. Marked increase in Means scores were demonstrated for trainees across all systems-professional status and educational levels.

A qualitative analysis of responses to one of the five critical incidents designed to measure trainees ability to utilize primary prevention on proposed intervention vs. traditional intervention indicates dramatic shift in response from pre-test to post-test. Thirty-nine trainees took pre-tests and post-tests which consisted of two components—program development and prevention skills. Practicum data showed that participation and practicum by County showed a far higher percentage of suburban and rural trainees who agreed to do a practicum as compared with urban. While a number of trainees who said that they would do a practicum was 80, only 25 completed it and 11 agencies were involved. Their years to continuing practicum was more work than expected, small amount of time restraints was the biggest one, another was work factors. Probably the practicum should have been introduced by the end of the first year if it were to have more impact. Trainee interview data indicated that case application increased markedly from year one to year two, use of tapes increased from 13% to 37%, inservice increased from 16% to 46%, and teaching from 14% to 37%.

Change of existing system showed the mental health system increased interest in staff development, more uniform sense of cooperation among people in the program, and psychiatric hospitals families included in planning patient care and working closer with community agencies. Education system showed emphasis on more inservicing and including values clarification and other prevention oriented topics in primary grades. In daycare, more emphasis was put on working with families and with special day care centers, looking in preventive terms to work with families. In the Health field, prevention concepts and skills included inservice and educational presentations at hospitals with more social service involvement in all units. The Obstetrics Department especially sought more mental health consultation with new mothers. Physicians gave more regular autopsy conferences to parents when an infant died which helped enhance the mourning. Liberalization in sibling visitation in maternity unit and policies of preparing children for the child's hospitalization were implemented. Drug and Alcohol Abuse Programs shifted to prevention rather than treatment. Social agencies working with child abuse showed an increased emphasis on prevention with families and an increased awareness of the effects of court placement of children. Academic professional schools of nursing implemented curriculum changes and showed more prevention in their curriculum.

Consumer satisfaction session evaluation and general program evaluations showed value in what was presented, the format of the presentations themselves, and the speakers. They liked the opportunity to meet these nationally famous people as well as the interaction with other professionals. Liked least were the topics, type of speakers, and desire for smaller groups of people at the sessions. The meetings were thought to be not too helpful by some of the trainees and some of the afternoon workshops did not seem to be topic-oriented and were somewhat disliked. It was found that the program did indeed result in increased knowledge and skills of prevention and its application training of all disciplines. Ninety-two% of the respondents stated a desire for a resource center and additional training programs.

Summary

The training program in primary prevention of childhood mental disorders has been successful in accomplishing program objectives of recruiting and maintaining a group of trainees from tri-county area with multidisciplinary backgrounds and from varied professional and educational levels.

The program has been successful in meeting original impact objectives—e.g., trainees demonstrate increase in knowledge and skills in primary prevention and have reported increased application of materials reported and documented development of primary prevention programs. Dissemination of materials has been accomplished. Future recommendations are: (a) that training programs in primary prevention could be most effectively directed toward caregivers from middle level administration and academic professional levels; (b) program design information and technical assistance should be provided earlier in the projects; and (c) future training projects suggested should provide shorter, more intensive programs for fewer trainees at a time.

REFERENCES

Bloom, B. PhD, *Prevention of Mental Disorders,* Community Mental Health Journal, Vol 15(3), 1979, pp. 179-191.
Caplan, G. *Prevention of Mental Disorders in Children,* New York Basic Books, Inc, 1961.

SOME ISSUES FROM THE FEDERAL VANTAGE POINT*

Thomas F. A. Plaut, PhD

ABSTRACT. Mental health promotion and mental illness prevention activities at the Federal level are viewed in the context of recent developments in both mental health and general health. Different target groups for such programs are listed as are different "levels" of prevention. The adequacy of the current knowledge base for prevention work is reviewed. Finally, basic principles underlying the current prevention/promotion activities of the National Institute of Mental Health are presented.

Background

Although recent interest in prevention has been stimulated by the Report of the President Commission on Mental Health (Report to the President, Vol I, 1978) and the Mental Health Systems Act, the concept of prevention in the mental health/mental illness area is not new. Gerald Caplan, for example, outlined many of the issues in his writing over fifteen years ago (Caplan, 1964). In the general health and medical care field there has been an analogous increased emphasis on prevention. In 1974 the Canadian Minister of Health, in the "LaLonde Report" (LaLonde, 1974) suggested

Thomas F. A. Plaut, PhD, MPH, is Special Assistant to the Director, National Institute of Mental Health, Department of Health and Human Services, 5600 Fishers Lane, Room 11-103, Rockville, MD 20857.

*Views expressed herein are those of the author and do not necessarily reflect the opinions, official policies, or position of the National Institute of Mental Health.

that the only practical means of achieving any significant reduction in rates of mortality (death) or morbidity (illness/disability) was through modification of persons' life styles. "Life styles" includes nutrition, exercise, and other health-related behavior such as smoking, drug and alcohol use, driving, use of firearms, and management of stress. In a comparable report issued by the Surgeon General of the U.S. Public Health Service (Healthy People, 1979) comparable strategies are outlined for improving the health of Americans.

The Report of the President's Commission (Report to the President, 1978) entitled one of its eight major recommendation chapters, "A Strategy for Prevention." There had been no such emphasis on this area in the report of the 1960 mental health commission (Action for Mental Health, 1961). The President's Commission made three recommendations in relation to the National Institute of Mental Health (NIMH): (1) that NIMH establish a Center on Prevention, (2) that primary prevention be the major activity of this Center, and (3) that ten million dollars be immediately appropriated for prevention with a ten year goal of 10% of the total NIMH budget being committed to this area. In 1979 NIMH established an Office on Prevention and in the fall of that year the Alcohol, Drug Abuse and Mental Health Administration of the Department of Health and Human Services organized a major conference on prevention (Proceedings, 1980). Even prior to this time NIMH had undertaken significant prevention activities under the leadership of Steve Goldston; i.e. the publication of *Primary Prevention: An Idea Whose Time has Come* (Klein and Goldston, 1977) and initiation of an NIMH Primary Prevention Series.

In 1980, using the first Congressional appropriation of earmarked prevention research funds ($4,000,000) NIMH awarded special research grants in two areas related to "children at risk." The first set of projects focused on research related to interventions seeking to assist children from disrupted families (divorce/separation) and the second focused on children of severely disturbed parents (mentally ill, alcoholic, or drug abusers).

Section 208 of the Mental Health Systems Act authorizes funds for a range of preventive activities. This law, however, does not become effective until October 1981. The extent of implementation of this section will depend on appropriation action by the Congress. The Systems Act also requires NIMH to establish an administrative unit dealing with prevention.

At the local level many community mental health centers have developed primary prevention activities as part of their consultation and education programs. Over the last ten years a number of states have established prevention units within the State Mental Health agencies—in 1980 at least eight states had such a unit. The first issue of the *Journal of Prevention* appeared—with an editorial board of nationally-known experts.

The term ''primary prevention'' has long been used in the field of public health. It refers to activities focusing on reducing the occurrence of new cases of a disease or illness. In the mental health field primary preventive activities are those directed at persons who do not exhibit any identifiable symptoms, i.e., are not psychiatrically ill.

Targets of Prevention/Promotion Activities

Prevention/promotion activities can be directed at a variety of different categories of persons or groups. The failure to specify the particular population which is being focused on often results in confusion and inadequate communication. Below are listed five ''classes'' or kinds of target populations for mental health promotion/mental illness prevention activities:

1. Persons ''at risk'' for major mental illness (schizophrenia or manic depressive disorders).
2. Persons ''at risk'' for other clearly defined ''mental conditions'' as specified in the Diagnostic Manual (Diagnostic and Statistical Manual, 1980).
3. Persons vulnerable to moderate anxiety or depression (but not necessarily diagnosable as ''psychiatrically ill'').
4. Children ''at risk'' for ''developmental attrition,'' a blockage of normal development (Eisenberg and Parron, 1979).
5. Persons with inadequate coping and/or persons who have not realized their full potentialities, generally the target of mental health promotion activities.

Some approaches are not directed specifically at any of the above categories of persons: Rather they emphasize the non-specific consequences of interventions. The underlying assumption here is that life circumstances, life events and crises increase vulnerability to a number of different mental and physical disorders. This type of intervention strategy (Bloom, 1979) moves away sharply from past approaches which emphasized identifiable etiological factors in a single illness.

Types of Interventions

Prevention/promotion activities also can vary in the level at which they are focused—individual, group, community, or institutional. While most preventive programs expect eventually to impact on individuals, a variety of intervening or mediating structures, groups, or organizations may be involved.

Some preventive interventions are directly focused on individuals, for example, teaching people better ways of coping with stress, improving cognitive problem-solving skills, anticipatory guidance to parents of seriously ill children, etc. Other preventive approaches focus on small (generally face-to-face) groups, including, but not restricted to, the family. Mental health preventive efforts can also be focused at the neighborhood or community level. An example is strengthening the role of "natural helpers" and increasing their utilization. Thus, an important mental health spin-off from a community-wide clean-up campaign may be the breaking down of communication barriers between neighbors. This may also increase the likelihood of the establishment of informal support (helping) networks that will be available to people when they are under stress or in crisis.

Institutional changes, at both micro and macro levels, constitute the last level of preventive interventions. "Micro" systems as used here, refers to local school systems, correctional systems, medical and health care institutions, day care centers, etc. The objective is to bring about changes in the ways in which these organizations operate so that they are more likely to promote mental health and less likely to be deleterious to the psychological health of the individuals and families who are their natural clientele. For example, for years parents of young children were not allowed any long visiting periods on the pediatric wards of hospitals. The rationale was that the children would be upset and tearful when their parents left and this was difficult for the hospital staff to deal with. In recent years it has increasingly been recognized that for most youngsters there is less of a sense of desertion and abandonment when parents visit regularly and for more than brief periods than was the case under prior policies.

"Macro" institutional change refers to modifications in the larger society, i.e., reduction of racism or sexism, income redistribution, modification of attitudes towards death or drug and alcohol use. Bringing about such large scale societal changes, while it may well carry promise of a "mentally healthier" society, is not generally viewed, however, as the responsibility of mental health agencies and professionals.

Adequacy of Knowledge Base

Probably the most frequently raised question about mental illness prevention and mental health promotion activities is: "Do we have enough knowledge to undertake preventive efforts?" There clearly is no consensus on the answer to this question. For example, Eisenberg (1977) and Lamb and Zussman (1979) doubt whether there is an adequate research base. On the other hand, in Volume IV of the Report of the President's Commission (1978) the Task Force on prevention presents a generally optimistic view of the current knowledge base. To some it appears that a "doublestandard" is being applied in relation to the adequacy of the knowledge base for action. That is, more evidence regarding effectiveness seems to be required before preventive programs are supported than is the case for treatment activities. In American society, generally there is greater public demand to "do something" when a person is ill or suffering than to undertake preventive efforts. Prevention is accepted in principle, but when hard resources allocation choices are made, the decision usually goes for treatment services. The White House Office on Science and Technology has recently estimated that no more than 15% of generally accepted medical technology (surgery, pharmacological treatments, and so on) have been fully evaluated and found to be effective and safe (Klerman, 1979).

Principles Underlying the NIMH Prevention Program

Although the NIMH prevention program was not formally established until 1979, a number of principles can be identified. Five of these principles are:

1. Priority to primary prevention efforts, but some attention also to secondary prevention. The bulk of available resources will be directed to the primary prevention area, but some funds will also be set aside for secondary prevention activities. Secondary prevention activities would include studies of how to improve the early identification (case-finding) skills of various care-givers. These would include, but not be restricted to, non-psychiatric physicians. Promotion approaches in the mental health field will also be part of the work—including, but not restricted to, traditional health and public education.

2. Emphasis on knowledge development. Accent is being placed on the development of new knowledge and the careful testing and evaluation of all services and services demonstration programs. This is in contrast to an approach that would emphasize wide-scale dissemination of essentially

untested programs and substantial support of ongoing or proposed community-based service programs.

3. Major effort to collaborate with and utilize other components of the Department of Health and Human Services. The NIMH Office of Prevention is committed to working intensively with other relevant components of the Institute—research, services, training, and education. This approach also applies to cooperative efforts with other components of the Public Health Services and other units in the Department, such as the Office of Human Development and the Center for Disease Control. In each case, existing programs within the Department will be examined to see what opportunities they present for mental illness prevention/mental health promotion activities. The newly developing area of behavioral medicine presents unusual opportunities for bridge-building with the mental health field. An example of this is the interest in stress which cuts across the NIMH and the "categorical" disease Institutes within the National Institutes of Health (cancer, heart disease, etc.)

4. Utilizing limited federal resources for "capacity-building purposes." It appears unlikely that large-scale Federal funds will be available for mental health promotion/mental illness prevention activities in the foreseeable future. The approach then will be to use the limited funds that are appropriated (for example, under the Mental Health Systems Act) to strengthen the capacity of existing general mental health programs—particularly at state levels—to provide effective leadership for the planning, development, and implementation of preventive work at both state and community levels.

5. Planned strategy to improve quality of work in the prevention area. Central to the program philosophy is attracting highly competent workers throughout the U.S. to the research, training, and action (services) aspects of prevention work. The objective is to "legitimate" (and make attractive) this area for quality scientific and other professional endeavors. The goal, then, is to get prevention "on the agenda" of many groups organizations and institutions. A major method for achieving this objective is the building of linkages among previously unrelated individuals or groups; the establishment of networks among researchers, among training institutions, among services personnel, and between all three of these groups.

REFERENCES

Action for Mental health. Report of the Joint Commission on Mental Illness and Health, New York, Basic Books, 1961.

Bloom, B.L. Prevention of mental disorders: Recent advances in theory and practice. *Community Mental Health Journal,* 1979, *15*(3); 179-191.

Caplan, G. *Principles of preventive psychiatry*. New York, Basic Books, 1964.

Diagnostic and Statistical Manual of Mental Disorders (3rd ed.) Washington, D.C. American Psychiatric Association, 1980.

Eisenberg, L. The perils of prevention: A cautionary note. *New England Journal of Medicine*. 1977, *297;* 1230-32.

Eisenberg, L. & Parron, D. Strategies for the prevention of mental disorders. *Healthy people: The surgeon general's report on health promotion and disease prevention, background papers*. (DHEW PHS Pub. No. 79-55071A), Washington, D.C., U.S. Government Printing Office, 1979, 135-155.

Healthy people: The surgeon general's report on health promotion and disease prevention, (DHEW PHS Pub. No. 79-55071). Washington, D.C.: U.S. government Printing Office, 1979.

Klein, D. C. & Goldston, S.E. (Eds.). *Primary prevention: An idea whose time has come.* (DHEW PHS Pub. No. (ADM) 77-447). U.S. Government Printing Office, 1978.

Klerman, G.L. Report to the National Advisory Mental Health Council, December, 1979, unpublished.

Lalonde, M. *A new perspective on the health of Canadians*. Ottawa, Canada, Government of Canada, 1974.

Lamb, H.R. & Zusman, J. Primary prevention in perspective. *American Journal of Psychiatry,* 1979, *136;* 12-17.

Proceedings- first annual conference on prevention, the Alcohol, Drug Abuse, and Mental Health Administration (DHEW ADM) Washington, D.C., U.S. Government Printing Office, in press, 1980.

Report to the President from the President's Commission on Mental Health, Volume I (Stock Number 040-000-00390-8). Washington, D.C.: U.S. Government Printing Office, 1978.

Report to the President from the President's Commission on Mental Health, Vol IV (Stock Number 040-000-0393-2). Washington, D.C.: U.S. Government Printing Office, 1978.

PRIMARY PREVENTION:
AN ANNOTATED BIBLIOGRAPHY

Susan Meehan

Programs for Early Childhood

Allen, George J., Chinsky, Jack M., Larcen, Stephen W., Lochman, John E., & Selinger, Howard V. *Community psychology and the schools: A behaviorally oriented multilevel preventive approach.* Hillsdale, New Jersey: Lawrence Erlbaum, 1976. Describes a program that incorporates a three-level intervention program within a school system to improve their interpersonal functioning. Discusses both theoretical background and practical operation.

Anthony, E. James. Primary prevention with school children. In Barten, Harvey H., & Bellak, Leopold (Eds.) *Progress in community mental health: Volume II.* New York: Grune & Stratton, 1972. Discusses the school as a setting for primary prevention in the development of children under conditions of psychiatric risk.

Blumberg, Marvin L. Character disorders in traumatized and handicapped children. *American Journal of Psychotherapy,* 1979, *33,* 201–213. Innate disabilities of physically handicapped and mentally retarded chil-

Susan Meehan received her BS degree from the Program in Child Development and Child Care, School of Health Related Professions, University of Pittsburgh, Pittsburgh, Pennsylvania in April 1981. Requests for reprints may be sent to the author at RD #4, McDonald, PA 15057.

dren predispose them to abuse or neglect by the family or social environment stresses, resulting in character disorders. Early multidisciplinary preventive interventions are discussed.

Blumberg, Marvin L. Prophylactic psychotherapy with children. *American Journal of Psychotherapy*, 1973, *27*, 155–165. Discusses the need of prophylactic psychotherapy at various stages of emotional and cognitive development for the prevention of psychopathology in otherwise emotionally healthy children.

Bolman, William M. An outline of preventive psychiatric programs for children. *Archives of General Psychiatry*, 1967, *17*, 5–8. Describes approaches to community-based prevention programs for children in terms of target populations, program goals, program types, and available resources.

Bower, Eli M. K.I.S.S. and kids: A mandate for prevention. *American Journal of Orthopsychiatry*, 1972, *42*, 556–565. Describes the use of four basic functions—health services, families, peer-play arrangements, and school as an alternative for the use of primary prevention.

Bronfenbrenner, Urie. Is early intervention effective? *Day Care and Early Education*, 1974, *2*, 15–19. Presents summarized research results of different intervention programs, some principles of early intervention that appear essential for effective programs, and stages of intervention from preparation for parenthood to ages six through twelve.

Caplan, Gerald. Opportunities for school psychologists in the primary prevention of mental disorders in children. *Mental Hygiene*, 1963, *47*, 525–539. Describes primary prevention and implications for its use in schools, including identification of crises and the role of school psychologists.

Caplan, Gerald (Ed.). *Prevention of mental disorders in children.* New York: Basic Books, Inc., 1961. Explores ideas of some pioneers in research concerning preventive psychiatry for children.

Cary, Ara C., & Reveal, Mary T. Prevention and detection of emotional disturbances in preschool children. *American Journal of Orthopsychiatry*, 1967, *37*, 719–724. Describes a program of nursery school and mother-group-guidance to provide an opportunity for prevention and case finding.

Friedrich, M. P. H., & Boriskin, Jerry A. Primary prevention of child abuse: Focus on the special child. *Hospital & Community Psychiatry,* 1978, *29,* 248–251. Review of literature on child abuse and present evidence that premature, sickly, or handicapped children are at high risk for abuse. Methods of identification and primary prevention to reduce parental stress and help prevent child abuse are discussed.

Hanson, Marci J., & Bellamy, G. Thomas. Continuous measurement of progress in infant intervention programs. *Education and Training of the Mentally Retarded,* 1977, *12,* 52–58. Supports the use of a continuous measurement strategy to assess the effects of and facilitate intervention programs. Focuses on a Down's Syndrome population with parents as intervention agents.

Harrison, Saul I., & Delano, James G. The status of prevention in the education of child psychiatrists. *Child Psychiatry and Human Development,* 1976, *7,* 3–21. Discusses results of a survey of child psychiatric residency programs suggesting that education in prevention is minimal and ambiguous. Followed by suggestions for child psychiatric education.

Kraft, Ivor. Preventing mental ill health in early childhood. *Mental Hygiene,* 1964, *48,* 413–423. Primary prevention is viewed as an aspect of social medicine or sociology and social work.

Lapides, Joseph. The school psychologist and early education: An ecological view. *Journal of School Psychology,* 1977, *15,* 184–189. Presents ecological perspective of psychological services to preschool children as a proactive delivery system concentrating on prophylactic activity.

Long, Barbara Ellis. A model for elementary school behavioral science as an agent of primary prevention. *American Psychologist,* 1970, *25,* 571–574. Gives a program based on a socioeducational model in behavioral sciences that is useful for primary prevention.

Newton, M.R., & Brown, Racine D. A preventive approach to developmental problems in school children. In Bower, Eli M., and Hollister,

William G. *Behavioral science frontiers in education.* New York: John Wiley & Sons, Inc., 1967. Presents models of intervention frequently used in dealing with school-age stress and crisis, then gives prevention program used by authors in South Carolina school. Program consisted of pre-school parent and child interviews, summer activities, individualized preparation for school entry and consultative collaboration with the classroom teacher.

Peterson, William D., & Nelson, Richard C. Helping children to cope with death. *Elementary School Guidance and Counseling,* 1975, *9,* 226–232. Discusses preparing children to deal with death of relatives or friends as a primary prevention measure against later problems in dealing with it.

Resch, Ruth C., Lilleskov, Roy K., Schur, Helen M., & Mihalov, Thelma. Infant day care as a treatment intervention: A follow-up comparison study. *Child Psychiatry and Human Development,* 1977, *7,* 147–155. Compares and evaluates differences between 3-year old children who had been in an infant day care treatment program and matched normal children who were entering regular day care for the first time.

Roen, Sheldon R. Primary prevention in the classroom through a teaching program in the behavioral sciences. In Cowen, Emory L., Gardner, Elmer A., & Zax, Melvin (eds.) *Emergent approaches to mental health problems.* New York: Appleton-Century-Crofts, 1967. Describes two approaches used for primary prevention in the classroom, as well as a specific behavioral sciences curriculum and ideas for further implementation of such programs.

Zax, Melvin et al. A teacher-aide program for preventing emotional disturbances in young schoolchildren. *Mental Hygiene,* 1966, *50,* 406–415. Details a program of primary prevention using the interpersonal skills of aides to help children remain in the mainstream of class routine.

Parent/Family Programs

Beebe, E. Rick. Expectant parent classes: A case study. *The Family Coordinator,* 1978, *27,* 55–58. Describes primary prevention program called Expectant Parent Program in Pennsylvania in terms of development, content, staff, and funding. Reviews some of the results of evaluation by involved parents. Provides a model for education to increase the effectiveness of parenting.

Berlin, Irving N., & Berlin, Roxie. Parents role in education as primary prevention. Paper presented at the Fiftieth Annual Meeting of the American Orthopsychiatric Association. New York City, May 1973. Describes data from several pilot projects and gives rationale for a prevention program benefiting mental health of both children and their parents.

Berlin, Roxie, & Berlin, Irving N. Parents' advocate role in education as primary prevention. In Berlin, Irving N. (Ed.) *Advocacy for child mental health.* New York: Brunner/Mazel, 1975. Discusses the use of parent involvement in children's education to enhance the child's and parent's feelings of being effective, and contributing to positive mental health.

Kane, Ruth P. The family's role in primary prevention. *Journal of Children in Contemporary Society,* 1981, *14*(2/3). Defines primary prevention, and discusses its roles in family therapy.

Kern, Joseph C., Tippman, Joan, Fortgang, Jeffrey, & Paul, Stewart R. A treatment approach for children of alcoholics. *Journal of Drug Education,* 1977-78, *7,* 207-218. Details sessions designed in an effort of education and prevention with children of alcoholics and their mothers to avoid second generation occurrences. Recommendations for programming of this type are also offered.

Lieberman, E. James. Preventive psychiatry and family planning. *Journal of Marriage and the Family,* 1964, *26,* 471-477. Based on the circular relationship between excess fertility and the conditions of poverty and its relevance for preventive psychiatry.

Morris, Marian G., Gould, Robert W., & Matthews, Patricia J. Toward prevention of child abuse. *Children,* 1964, *11,* 55-60. Presents consistent social signs which have implications for early identification of neglectful or abusive parents and for prevention of further neglect and abuse.

Polak, Paul R., Egan, Donald, Vandenbergh, Richard, Williams, W. Vail. Prevention in mental health: A controlled study. *American Journal of Psychiatry,* 1975, *132,* 146–149. Families who had experienced a sudden death of a member were given crisis intervention services. Results of the study were not supportive of the hypothesis that such services decrease the risk of psychiatric illness. Discusses rationale for these findings.

Signell, Karen A. Kindergarten entry: A preventive approach to community mental health. *Community Mental Health Journal,* 1972, *8,* 60–70. A model program using small group discussions with parents at kindergarten entry time. The aim was education for a population with a long-range goal of training mothers as mental health resources for the community.

Signell, Karen A. On a shoestring: A consumer-based source of personpower for mental health education. *Community Mental Health Journal,* 1976, *12,* 342–354. Describes how mental health professionals can start a consumer-based primary prevention program by teaching nonprofessionals, such as parents, their skills. Reports results of research on effectiveness of such a program.

General Theories, Viewpoints, Programs

Albee, George W., & Joffe, Justin M. *Primary prevention of psychopathology.* Hanover, New Hampshire: University Press of New England, 1977. Leaders in the field present a diversity of views and approaches to the subject of primary prevention.

Arsenian, John. Toward prevention of mental illness in the United States. *Community Mental Health Journal,* 1965, *1,* 320–325. Identifies major sources of tension, and outlines some approaches for reducing the aspects of experience which generate this tension and presumably bear on the incidence of mental illness.

Bolman, William M., & Westman, Jack C. Prevention of mental disorder: An overview of current programs. *American Journal of Psychiatry,* 1967, *123,* 1058–1068. Presents current techniques and programs for the prevention of mental disorder, including child-centered, family-centered, and society-centered preventions.

Bower, Eli M. Primary prevention of mental and emotional disorders: A conceptual framework and action possibilities. *American Journal of Orthopsychiatry,* 1963, *33,* 832–848. Presentation and discussion of a conceptualization of primary prevention, and programs of research and demonstration.

Broskowski, Anthony & Baker, Frank. Professional, organizational, and social barriers to primary prevention. *American Journal of Orthopsychiatry,* 1974, *44,* 707–719. Develops a comprehensive view of the professional, organizational, and social barriers to the design, development, and implementation of primary prevention programs.

Caplan, Gerald. *Principles of preventive psychiatry.* New York: Basic Books, 1964. Addressed to a wide range of mental health workers, this book provides a model for primary prevention, as well as presenting a theory of community mental health practice and a discussion of methods of such preventive psychiatry.

Chalke, F. C. R., & Day, J. J. (Eds.). *Primary prevention of psychiatric disorders.* Toronto: University of Toronto Press, 1968. Discusses the development, role, and future of primary prevention as well as the medical aspects and methods for usage.

Cherniss, Cary. Creating new consultation programs in community mental health centers: Analysis of a case study. *Community Mental Health Journal,* 1977, *13,* 133–141. Presents rationale for the failure of a primary prevention program initiated in a community mental health center to become fully operational. Presents recommendations for such programs.

Cumming, Elaine. Primary prevention—more cost than benefit. In Gottesfeld, Harry. *The critical issues of community mental health.* New York: Behavioral Publications, 1972. Based on issues of the lack of tests of the effectiveness of primary prevention strategies, the removal of needed manpower from the treatment of the mentally ill caused by such strategies, and the attack of moral and social problems because of their insupportability rather than their being the cause of mental illness.

Dorr, Darwin. An ounce of prevention. *Mental Hygiene,* 1972, *56,* 25–27. Discusses the high costs of community health programs and the resultant savings of these primary prevention programs.

Flanagan, John C. Evaluation and validation of research data in primary prevention. *American Journal of Orthopsychiatry,* 1971, *41,* 117–123. Treats each of five factors in validating research related to primary prevention studies in order to review some problems of primary prevention research data and summarize the procedures for the results to be considered valid.

Forgays, Donald G. (Ed.). *Primary prevention of psychopathology. Vol. 2.* Hanover, New Hampshire: University Press of New England, 1978. Theme of environmental factors contributing to the development of psychopathology, and environmental manipulations which may effectively prevent psychopathology.

Garmezy, Norman. Vulnerability research and the issue of primary prevention. *American Journal of Orthopsychiatry,* 1971, *41,* 101–117. Discusses a strategy for determining vulnerability information which is needed to achieve primary prevention.

Kelly, James G. The quest for valid preventive interventions. In Rosenblum, Gershen (Ed.), *Issues in community psychology and preventive mental health.* New York: Behavioral Publications, 1971. Presents three contrasting approaches for preventive interventions which suggest new criteria for change in programs.

Kelly, James G. Toward an ecological conception of preventive interventions. In Carter, J. W. (Ed.) *Research contributions from psychology to community mental health.* New York: Behavioral Publications, Inc., 1968. Describes preventive interventions designed for two types of high schools based upon the knowledge of ecological principles and adapting social environments.

Kessler, Mark, & Albee, George W. Primary prevention. *Annual Review of Psychology,* 1975, *26,* 557–591. Definitions, important target models, epidemiology, and social conflicts involved with primary prevention. Points out where efforts are being made and what the future may hold. Discusses difficulties for scientific study and research problems.

Kiesler, Frank. Programming for prevention. *North Carolina Journal of Mental Health,* 1965, *1,* 3–17. Describes method of programming for a community mental health program. Includes graph on professional distribution and groundwork rules.

Klein, Donald C., & Goldston, Stephen E. (Eds.). *Primary prevention: An idea whose time has come.* Washington, D.C.: U.S. Government Printing Office, 1977. DHEW Publication No. (ADM) 77-447. Proceedings of a pilot conference held April 2-4, 1976 sponsored by NIMH and NAMH. Discusses primary prevention for specific target groups, agency strategies, and aspects of prevention.

McCord, Joan. A thirty-year follow-up of treatment effects. *American Psychologist,* 1978, *33,* 284-289. Treatment program for over 250 men because of delinquency-prediction scores is indicated to have negative side effects. Discusses possible explanations for these findings.

Mitchell, David C., & Scherman, Avraham. The other side of the mountain. *Journal of Clinical Child Psychology,* 1977, *6,* 30-31. Presents an argumentive proposal for primary prevention as an alternative mode of psychological intervention. Defines primary prevention theoretically, as well as in the form of an applied community-based program & provides specific recommendations for the needed further research.

Ojemann, Ralph H. (Ed.). *Four basic aspects of preventive psychiatry.* Iowa: State University of Iowa, 1957. Preventive psychiatry in terms of its conceptualization, the factors associated with mental illness, recent research on education, and the future in research.

Perlmutter, Felice D., Vayda, Andrea M., & Woodburn, Paul K. An instrument for differentiating programs in prevention - primary, secondary, and tertiary. *American Journal of Orthopsychiatry,* 1976, *46,* 533-541. Discusses an instrument developed to identify critical dimensions in consideration for differentiating among prevention programs, and to help define the complex issues underlying the design of such programs. Based on the concept that prevention is not adequately understood by practitioners in the field, and so has not become a major component of mental health programs.

Poser, Ernest G., & King, Michael C. Primary prevention of fear: An experimental approach. In Sarason, Irwin G., & Spielberger, Charles

D. (Eds.) *Stress and anxiety: Volume 3*. New York: John Wiley & Sons, 1976. Explores different approaches to primary prevention and reviews studies from other investigators.

Raphael, Beverley. Preventive intervention with the recently bereaved. *Archives of General Psychiatry*, 1977, *34*, 1450-1454. Study of the effectiveness of preventive intervention in lowering postbereavement morbidity.

Sauber, S. Richard. *Preventive educational intervention for mental health*. Cambridge: Ballinger Publishing Company, 1973. Theoretical and practical foundations for preventive mental health educational intervention. Includes many figures, tables, and appendix items. Discusses basic concepts, education for community service personnel, possibilities and problems, a working concept, and evaluation methods.

Schecter, Marshall D. Prevention in psychiatry—problems and prospects. *Child Psychiatry and Human Development*, 1970, *1*, 68-82. Discusses the consideration of the use of preventive modes on the basis of the correlation between genetic, intrauterine, environmental, and interactive factors.

Signell, Karen A. Training nonprofessionals as community instructors: A mental health education model of primary prevention. *Journal of Community Psychology*, 1975, *3*, 365-373. Describes effective processes in training nonprofessionals for giving communication courses and other mental health education work in the community as a mode of primary prevention.

Silverman, Phyllis Rolfe. Services to the widowed: First steps in a program of preventive intervention. *Community Mental Health Journal*, 1967, *3*, 37-44. Widowed people under the age of 60 have a high risk of becoming mentally ill. Describes phases of bereavement, and relates them to existing preventive services administered in the study. Preventive measures for mental health agencies and other caregivers are also discussed.

Symposium on preventive and social psychiatry. Washington, D.C.: Walter Reed Army Institute of Research, 1957. Six sessions, each session dealing with human group problems from overlapping but different points of view.

VanAntwerp, Malin. The route to primary prevention. *Community Mental Health Journal,* 1971, *7,* 183-188. Describes the place of primary prevention as it exists, gives reasons why the nation has hesitated to move into primary prevention, and provides new information on which to form a primary prevention strategy.

Visotsky, Harold M. Primary prevention. In Freedman, Alfred M., Kaplan, Harold I. (Eds.). *Comprehensive textbook of psychiatry.* Baltimore: The Williams & Wilkins Company, 1967. Describes the concept of primary prevention as well as the role of institutions of society in the use of primary prevention techniques.

Wagenfeld, Morton O. The primary prevention of mental illness: A sociological perspective. *Journal of Health & Social Behavior,* 1972, *13,* 195-203. Examines the nature of and evidence concerning primary prevention.

DATE DUE

MAY 3 0 1989		
JUL 1 0 1995		
APR 0 1 1996		

DEMCO 38-297